The Sociology of Health

STUDIES IN SOCIOLOGY

Consulting Editor, CHARLES H. PAGE
UNIVERSITY OF MASSACHUSETTS

The Sociology
of Health:

An Introduction

ROBERT N. WILSON

School of Public Health,
UNIVERSITY OF NORTH CAROLINA

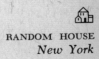

RANDOM HOUSE
New York

98

To
    John C. Cassel,
    social physician

Preface

This book is the outgrowth of several years' experience in medical sociology and public health and is designed as a brief introduction to certain salient issues in the field. It is written from the stance of a behavioral scientist who construes human health as a topic both of inherent theoretical interest to the curious sociologist and of compelling pragmatic importance to all who care about man's ability to live to capacity. The treatment itself is in the form of a preface or first statement. It is neither a comprehensive text nor an exploration of any single facet of social medicine in depth. Rather, it is an attempt to say, "Here is how the field looks to me, and these are some of the themes that seem to bear the prospect of intellectual excitement and humane involvement."

R. N. W.

Acknowledgments

Because I have been employed intermittently in the field of medical sociology during the past seventeen years, it is manifestly impossible to trace the congeries of influence with much assurance. Among my formal teachers, Talcott Parsons, Henry A. Murray, and George C. Homans were the heaviest shapers, although I doubt that any of them would be eager to confess that the current product meets his design specifications.

My service in the ranks of medical sociologists does fall into four distinct periods, and the colleagues with whom I worked at each juncture have been willing tutors. At Cornell, from 1951 to 1953, I was introduced to the study of medical organization by Temple Burling and Edith M. Lentz in a happy collaboration that eventuated in *The Give and Take in Hospitals* (New York: Putnam, 1956). With the Social Science Research Council in 1955 and 1956, I had the good fortune to work with the council's Committee on Social Psychiatry. There I enjoyed an especially close association with John A. Clausen and Alexander H. Leighton, which centered around our editorship of *Explorations in Social Psychiatry* (New York: Basic Books, 1957). From 1957 to 1960, at the Harvard Medical School and the Department of Social Relations, Robert N. Rapoport and I joined in responsibility for the Training Program for Social Scientists in Medicine. Many of the ideas in this book grew in our continuing seminar of those years and were first elaborated in an unpublished manuscript that Dr. Rapoport and I wrote and edited under partial support by the Russell Sage Foundation. I am especially grateful to him for permission to draw on that manuscript.

Since 1963, while on the faculty of the School of Public Health at the University of North Carolina, I have learned a great deal from colleagues, both health professionals and social scientists. In particular, I should like to thank John C. Cassel, Herman A. Tyroler, C. David Jenkins, Ralph C. Patrick, Jr., Cecil Slome, John T. Fulton, and Berton H. Kaplan for their wisdom and encouragement. My debt to these scholars in Chapters 5 through 8 will be especially evident to them.

Finally, it is a pleasure to acknowledge the secretarial and editorial assistance of Natalie Harbin, a devoted co-worker.

Contents

Introduction

Medicine, of course, has always been recognized as a bio-social science and an interpersonal art. The history of medicine abounds in figures who viewed man's health and illness as inextricably woven together with the way man lives. From Hippocrates to Paracelsus to Rudolf Virchow to Sigmund Freud, wise physicians have been concerned with linking the individual's perception of himself and others, his whole experience of the social universe, to the efficacious or inept functioning of his bodily processes. Yet the study of social psychological features in the genesis of disease and the course of healing remained largely implicit and unsystematic until the early twentieth century. Why?

One reason, surely, for the relative neglect of medicine's social ties has been the long sequence of attempts to locate illness in some single property or entity that would constitute a final "cause." The humors and demons and substances that served explanatory purposes in ancient and medieval medical practice deflected attention from the normal round of life events. With the rise of scientific medicine in the nineteenth century, the enormously powerful germ theory of disease again drew observation away from the intrapersonal and interpersonal arena and fixed it upon the microorganism. And the germ theory *worked*. It was responsible for splendid triumphs over infectious and communicable diseases, for the rationale underlying complicated surgery, and for fresh comprehension of organic processes. It might, however, be asserted that the germ theory worked too well. The quest of causal "villains"—the specific germ attached to the specific disease entity—so captivated medical thinkers that they could spare little energy for other elements in the web of causation. This concentration on organic etiology proved insufficient when the health scene became increasingly characterized (as it is in our own day) by the prevalence of chronic, and especially mental, disorders.

A second major reason for the late emergence of a sophisticated social medicine was the underdeveloped state of the social sciences themselves. Although the sciences of human behavior are still at a very early stage, they have undergone substantial growth in knowledge and technique during the past fifty years. In their contribution to enhanced understanding of health and illness, the disciplines of anthropology, sociology, and psychology have been preeminent. Recently, economics and political science have begun to add heavily to our grasp of the patterns of medical care and the nature of societal response to health problems. The social sciences have reemphasized man's wholeness, his simultaneous existence as a biological, psychological, and social creature. Freud's influence has been especially powerful in relating aspects of mental life to the individual's total possibilities of functioning. Cultural anthropology has underlined the impress of group values and customs on personal behavior. Sociology has stressed the way in which styled currents of interpersonal relations generate repetitive modes of acting, notably including modes of illness and wellness. Today, the maturing social sciences are engaged in a flourishing interchange with medical science, an interchange that promises great benefits to both sets of disciplines, each set central to our understanding of human behavior in health and sickness.

This juncture of medicine and social science, often conveniently, if inaccurately, termed "medical sociology" (inaccurately, because many fields other than sociology are involved), has shown impressive growth, particularly in the United States, in the years since World War II. The major reasons for growth are probably, as sketched above, increased medical receptivity and increased social scientific competence. But these underlying themes have been brought to a quickened expression by the ready availability of men and money at this particular point in time. The pool of scientific manpower that could be devoted to medical-social concerns was enormously enlarged in the postwar years by the expansion of graduate studies in the social sciences. It is surely not accidental that the first thrust of recognizable numbers of young social scientists into health affairs coincided with the attainment of the doctorate by the first wave of research scholars who had been supported by the GI Bill after World War II. At just about the same period—the late 1940s and early 1950s—medical research, especially under the impetus of the National Institutes of Health, enjoyed relatively generous financial underpinning. Thus we experienced a fortuitous merger of patterns in which developing intellectual interests could be fairly swiftly translated into concrete research and teaching activities because the manpower and money were available.

Despite some faltering and misunderstanding and some superficial work that partook of the merely fashionable or opportunistic, this period of explosive growth has been, on the whole, salutary. The social sciences have become quite solidly built into the health enterprise, and the specialty of medical social science comprises one of the largest and most energetic subdisciplines within the sociological and psychological professions. Valuable contributions to medicine have been and are being made by social scientists, and in turn, the inquiring sociologist or anthropologist has found the health world a rich context for a variety of research interests.

Like all growth spurts, however, this one has been markedly uneven. Social science has offered more to research than to teaching. It has added more to the investigation of organizational and professional patterns than to inquiry into the fundamentals of disease etiology and therapy. Certain sectors of the medical enterprise—mental health, public health, and hospital administration—have been more warmly hospitable to behavioral studies than others—medical schools, internal medicine, and surgery. Further, one might contend that the involvement with medicine has been more beneficial to the social sciences themselves thus far as a source of data to test familiar ideas and as a generally enlightening interdisciplinary experience than as a source of substantial fresh theory or knowledge.

The collaboration between medical and social sciences will very likely widen and deepen in the latter decades of this century. To the internal pressures generated by emergent patterns in the disciplines themselves, such as the medical researcher's quest for social elements in the causes of chronic illness or the social psychologist's need for a sure grounding in the biology of behavior, are now added potent external pressures from a society that demands a more sophisticated and equitable distribution of health care. The imperative calls for new understanding of etiology, new modes of prevention and treatment, and new organization of care-giving processes; all these will tax the innovative capacities of those who work on the common frontier of health systems and social systems.

The substance of interaction between medicine and the social sciences includes a diverse range of topics, from hospital organization to therapeutic roles to the influence of psychological stress on patienthood. Roughly, however, this interplay may be grouped conveniently into the two main divisions suggested by Robert Straus of the University of Kentucky Medical Center: sociology *of* medicine and sociology *in* medicine. The distinction is not exact, and many activities overlap the two categories. Yet the bulk of professional concern may be characterized either as (1) detached observation and analysis, motivated primarily by a sense of *sociological* problem, or (2) more intimate, applied, and conjoint research and teaching, motivated primarily by a sense of *health* problem.

In its early stages, medical sociology was centered mainly in the first category. The initiation of social scientists into medical culture spurred them to examine health professionals and health institutions as novel objects of scientific curiosity. This disinterested (*not* uninterested) posture had important yields: a surer understanding of the professions, especially medicine and nursing; a better analysis of role relationships in the therapeutic encounter; and enhanced knowledge of the hospital's social structure. The view from the outside was not at all limited to increasing the social scientist's fund of data and ideas. It also had vital implications for the alignment of professional activities in the care of ill people.

Today, we discern what is perhaps more nearly an even balance of sociological effort. The student of society and personality is more and more often a regular member of the health enterprise in any of a number of capacities. He is full collaborator rather than detached observer, and he comes directly to grips with teaching, research, and service functions undertaken by health professionals. Indeed, the social scientist is regarded in many settings as being himself a variety of health professional, a colleague instead of an occasional consultant.

Although the distinction between outside analysis and inside partnership has been adopted as a useful organizing framework for this volume, it would be unfortunate to overstate the differences. The student of human behavior, like the poet, may be intrinsically a "doubled" man, alternately swimming within the steady current of affairs as a committed actor and meandering along the bank of the stream to chart the flow. He may be valuable in either guise.

In any event, the articulation of health sciences with social sciences appears likely to persist, and the number and density of connections will probably increase. Medicine is more clearly and more self-consciously part of society than ever before. The environing society, in turn, is ever more able to shift its attention from survival and subsistence to the cultivation of human possibilities, notably including the possibility of a healthful and fulfilling course of life.

PART ONE

From the Outside:
Sociology of Medicine

The sociology of medicine treats the medical world as an object of scientific curiosity. This approach is not geared primarily toward the solution of health problems, but rather toward an explanation of the behavior of physicians, patients, and nurses, and an understanding of the organizational structure in which they interact. Although the social scientist in this posture may illumine certain topics with important implications for practicing health professionals, his chief concern is understanding rather than action. Moreover, the structuring of problems typically derives from a sociological rather than a medical focus. For example, the social scientist sees hospitals as a species of bureaucratic organization or inter-professional role relationships, and compares them with other institutions such as the factory. He is not, in the first instance, devoted to discovering clues to more effective care for patients.

Hence Part One construes the sociologist as observer of health activities. In Part Two he will appear as much more nearly a collaborator in those activities, applying professional insight to the attack on the problems of illness in society.

CHAPTER 1

Defining Health
and Illness

A philosopher once remarked that "the problem of metaphysics is the problem of the categories." A similar statement could be made about every scientific field, indeed every intellectual discipline, because definition precedes sensible discussion, investigation, or action. All definitions demand consensus on the part of informed observers. This consensus is harder to achieve, however, in areas where "objective" yardsticks are few and human passions are at stake in the formulation. Each of these qualifications applies to health: medicine has no perfect meter, like the gold bar at Sèvres, to serve as a final criterion of judgment; nor do those who try to define the conditions of health ever find their discourse untouched by the fact that these phenomena engage men's deepest aspirations and fears. Not only does the variety of human behavior admit of many different categories for assigning healthiness or disease but also the question of who (the victim, the physican, the relative, or the formal agent of social control) is perceiving and defining becomes critical.

Physicians have traditionally held a rough, commonsensical view of health as "the absence of symptoms." Health therefore becomes a residual category, the uninteresting opposite of disease. However useful such a definition may be in separating the treatable and the classifiable from all others, it clearly begs several questions. It excludes from the category of illness the subtle and latent disturbance that has gone unremarked by the subject or is unapparent to the observer. By fixing attention on familiar signs of malfunction, the definition of health as nondisease also tends to exclude analysis of the well-functioning individual. We learn much about what is wrong but little about what is right, and thus we are enfeebled in efforts to prevent illness or to foster superior functioning. Finally, of course, symptoms themselves are rarely unambiguous: physicians may disagree on the appropriate scope or severity of symptoms for a given diagnosis, and many of the most important symptoms cannot be observed at all but must be inferred from the patient's report.

A radically different conception of health offered by one physician asserts that health is "compensated illness." Here the usual assumption is turned inside-out. Instead of positing health as the usual state of the human being and thinking of all illness as a deviation from some normal condition, this definition assumes that in a sense we are all ill and that our healthiness then represents an achievement in counteracting the incursions of disease. Among the attractive features of such a conception is its recognition of how pervasive illness, particularly chronic illness, is in contemporary societies and its implication that health is a process of living rather than a static entity. We do not, however, find in the idea of compensation any ready clues to severity or degree. How much compensation, one might ask, renders the person healthy?

Several approaches to the distinction between health and sickness are founded upon a conception of "normalcy," a state from which the deviations commonly leading to a classification of the individual as ill may be measured. The difficulty with gauging departures from the norm is that normalcy itself may take different guises. One obvious meaning of normal is the statistical idea that the normal is the average or most frequently occurring phenomenon. This interpretation is often of great value in medicine; the most conspicuous example is perhaps body temperature, where a fever can be quickly ascertained as a departure from a known average and is therefore a fairly reliable signal of disturbance. On the other hand, there are human groups in which conditions that medicine has clearly identified as pathology are endemic. Yaws, for example, has been found in some preliterate populations to be exhibited by the majority of individuals. In such a situation, few observers would be inclined to judge the sufferer from yaws healthy, even though persons free from the disease were statistically rarer than persons having it.

Another conception of normal takes the norm to be a model state of health, a standard to aim at that exceeds most peoples' current state of well-being. The norm as a realistically unattainable perfection has a provocative kinship with certain ideas about positive health or wellness. It, like the idea of health as compensated illness, represents superior functioning as an achievement whose attainment requires effort. If we take the normal to be a model, however, two important difficulties arise: we create an unmanageable and theoretically unwieldy category of abnormality or illness, such that we discern pathology at every turn, and we may set forth impossible criteria of health that are inappropriate to the bulk of usual life demands on individual capacity.

Still a third version of normalcy takes it to be neither the most frequent state of health nor the model of wellness but, rather, a condition of moderately effective functioning that shows no seriously disabling features. Here the emphasis is on the person as a "going concern" who is to be evaluated as healthy unless there are such severe derangements that the body system or the total behavioral repertoire or both are clearly inadequate to maintain the individual in his routine patterns of activity. By taking functional adequacy as a basic criterion, this approach makes it possible to link judgments about health to the social situations in which people find themselves. It admits, furthermore, of viewing health as a relative affair, so that individuals may be evaluated differentially and alternative healths are recognized, instead of a monolithic health standard to which all must repair.

The concept of health as functional efficacy enables the analyst to invoke considerations of appropriateness, of fitness for specified activities. That is, it begins to answer the question, Health for what? The health of a housewife is presumably quite different in some ways from the health of an actress; what is normally healthy in a twenty-year-old sprinter may be a state of functioning both impossible and undesirable in the middle-aged executive. If normal health consists of the ability to perform adequately in the individual's chief social roles, notably the familial and the occupational, then criteria of healthiness will vary as do the styled rights and obligations that form the substance of roles. Although American society (and most others) places a high value on health, effective functioning is not usually construed as an ultimate value, an end in itself. Health is cherished because of what it enables the person to do, and illness is feared primarily because of its interference with desired behaviors.

But, of course, the problem of defining health and illness is not only a question of trying to keep intellectual discourse clean and untrammeled. The concepts we adopt are intimately bound up in medical research, medical care, and eventually, in decisions about what levels of well-being a society will or will not tolerate. One observer has in fact argued that the field of public health advances through progressive redefinition of the unacceptable; a tolerable level of population health in 1900 may well be intolerable in 1970. Judgments about healthiness are therefore laced through the whole social fabric and affect everything from the individual's self-picture to the setting of national policy.

Much of our confusion in speaking sensibly about health is rooted in two characteristics of the phenomena: there are nearly always many parties to the definition rather than a single authoritative voice, and health itself is a complex of processes instead of a unified entity. At least three sources of evaluation are often present in deciding when an individual is ill: the person himself; other lay observers, such as relatives and friends; and the health professional. Social stability probably requires that the three coincide in the majority of instances, and serious difficulties arise when they are discrepant or when one of the parties is absent or unable to judge. The diversity of processes we identify as part of the domain of health may be readily seen in the familiar, if conceptually incorrect, separation between "physical," "psychological," and the recently added "social" functioning.

As we shall discuss in more detail in Chapter 2, different societies and various subsectors of a single society may hold importantly differing ideas about what constitutes health or illness. In part these various definitions rest on the range of conceptions about cause, so that illness or wellness comes to be linked to evidence regarding the individual's presumed exposure to some critical agent. Thus knowledge about the prevalence of germs—or the prevalence of witches—may determine judgments of illness. In part, too, variations of definition depend upon the differing functional demands placed upon persons occupying certain social roles in a given society. For instance, mild bronchitis may be a very serious illness to a professional singer and inconsequential to an executive. Low back pain that is merely an irritant to a salesman may be factually disabling to a dock worker.

In general, education and affluence tend to encourage stricter definition of health and decreased tolerance for the discomfort of illness. Cross-culturally, a similar trend may be noted: the developed industrial countries find poor health "unacceptable" at a lower threshold than do the developing rural countries. Membership in the higher strata of the social class system seems to entail a level of awareness about health possibilities that promotes a rigorous conception of wellness. The sources of this awareness are, first, sheer information, and second, the habit of mastery that people of high educational and occupational rank customarily bring to life's importunities. That is, middle and upper class individuals know more about the meaning of symptoms and the armamentarium of treatment; they come closest of any population groups to speaking the physician's language. Having recognized a health problem, they are then more disposed than other groups to define themselves as patients by seeking help, by striving to overcome the illness in full collaboration with medical professionals. Accompanying knowledge and the orientation to mastery, of course, historically has been and in large measure continues to be the ability to pay for care.

How different this posture toward illness is than the poignant outlook of a lower class respondent quoted by Earl L. Koos:

> I wish I really knew what you mean about being sick. Sometimes I've felt so bad I could curl up and die, but had to go on because the kids had to be taken care of, and besides, we didn't have the money to spend for the doctor—how could I be sick? . . . How do you know when you're sick, anyway? Some people can go to bed most any time with anything, but most of us can't be sick—even when we need to be.[1]

[1] Earl L. Koos, *The Health of Regionville* (New York: Columbia University Press, 1954), p. 30.

In recent years there have been a number of attempts to deal with the many facets of health/illness that may characterize a given individual and also to cope with the suggestion that health is a process, a sequence of behavior, rather than a fixed attribute of the person. It has been proposed, for example, that health be evaluated separately on at least three dimensions: organic, or physical, functioning; psychological functioning; and "social health," presumably identifying the individual's capacity to act in social roles. In such a scheme, ideal health—what Halbert Dunn called "high-level wellness"—would consist of maximizing people's position on all three measures, although with the realization that all individuals probably exhibit an unequal balance among them.

The notion that health and illness are dynamic patterns, changing with time and social circumstance, leads to the conclusion that judgments of healthiness must be made many times as the life history unfolds. It also pushes the analyst to reiterate that most evaluations of health are relative, based on a series of perceptions and observations rather than a unitary standard of measurement. Further, health comes in a dynamic framework to be seen as a continuum of functional ability-disability, finely graded, not as a matter of flat, mutually exclusive categories.

If we take "dis-ease" literally, as the lack or absence of ease, then we must of course ask, Whose ease? and In what context? Such questions seem especially relevant to the chronic illnesses, especially the mental disorders, which have assumed an increasingly important place in the contemporary United States. We have to assess functional capacity, and sentiments about that capacity, in the absence of classic clear-cut syndromes of disorder. Neurosis is different from typhoid fever, and rheumatoid arthritis is different from cholera. Therefore, we try to discover who it is that sees the subject as ill, and what purposes govern the act of labeling.

Fredrick C. Redlich [2] has commented that one operational definition of mental illness might be simply that a mentally ill

---

[2] Fredrick C. Redlich, "The Concept of Health in Psychiatry," in Alexander H. Leighton, John A. Clausen, and Robert N. Wilson (eds.), *Explorations in Social Psychiatry* (New York: Basic Books, 1957).

person is one who is in contact with a helping agent. An individual who has initiated a therapeutic relationship clearly fulfills at least several of the possible criteria for being judged as ill: he has so defined himself, he has presumably been so defined by a medical professional, and he has adopted the social role of a patient. On the other hand, if therapy were not self-initiated, the individual might be in contact with a helping agent at the behest of a relative or friend or under the suasion of legal agents, as in a court referral. He might in this instance fail to define himself as needing help and refuse to adopt the role of patient. We thus confront the issue of determining who has the power or influence to categorize another as ill and how nearly this labeler's evaluation must match the subject's own.

We have noted that in most cases the individual's subjective sense of illness or well-being is consonant with the judgments of health professionals and other concerned observers. The self-rating on number and severity of symptoms, for example, tends to agree quite well with the rating that would be derived from a physician's doing a thorough medical history and examination. Although portraying health in terms of Luigi Pirandello's version of reality would not be quite accurate, self-perception is crucial. To a major extent it is fair to say, "Healthy (or ill) you are if you think you are."

But self-perception does not stand alone and may in some situations be radically opposed to the way others perceive the subject. Evaluation of health from the outside is usually rooted in either or both of two kinds of judgment as to function: the non-performance of social roles or the distorted performance of them in a manner disturbing to the partner in the relationship or to interested third parties, such as the police or neighbors. Although each of these judgments may also be made by the individual himself, the second (role distortion) may be especially difficult for the subject to assess, and it would be especially vulnerable to varied interpretations on the part of the several participants in evaluation. Here again, the psychological disorders pose the gravest ambiguities of definition. This is partly because of their inherent complexity and partly because of the fact that role fulfillment is seldom an all-or-none proposition. What degree of incapacity must be present to merit the label of nonperformance?

How distorted must a given role relationship become before role partners affix the name of illness to the subject's vagaries of behavior?

If competence in role behavior is accepted as a primary criterion of health, then the process of definition is more emphatically a social process. And as we widen the perspective from the individual-as-entity to the individual's net of relationships with others, we may be forced to consider the vexed concept of "societal health" or group wellness. The health level of a population may be described in terms of rates of illness or disability. In this case, "group health" is merely the accumulation or summation of all the individual states of health composing the aggregate. When we analyze a community, however, we are dealing with a population whose members are related to one another in determinate ways. They are more than an aggregate. Hence, there may be reason to try to conceptualize the health behavior of a given group, or even of a total social system, as something other than the simple summation of individual health states.

The chief hazard in this sort of enterprise is, again, to discover agreement on criteria of social system health or group functional adequacy. One can assess an individual's ability to enact social roles, but how does one assess a community's functional "goodness"? A valiant effort in this area is the work of Alexander H. and Dorothea Leighton.[3] Although they do not speak directly of a concept of societal health, these investigators have attempted to link the occurrence of psychiatric symptoms to the nature of social relationships in the communities where the populations surveyed lived. The Leightons hypothesized that disorganized or poorly integrated communities would be associated with higher levels of population symptomatology than would well-organized communities. Their criteria for community integration were such factors as leadership patterns, the tenor of interpersonal relations, and the level of involvement in formal organizations. Communities judged to be well integrated did tend to exhibit lesser symptom levels, so that there is some reason to believe that societal health thus measured is positively connected to the health states of its participants singly considered.

As we enlarge our conception of health to embrace group

[3] Alexander H. Leighton, *My Name Is Legion* (New York: Basic Books, 1959).

relationships as well as the functional processes of the individual, we run into the danger of giving a limitless mandate to the health professional. If, logically, "all" of life, the total human universe, should come under his purview, this universe, nevertheless, is far from being his exclusive property. Thus the judgment of a physician that certain patterns of community organization are "healthier" than others must be tempered by the realization that social health on his terms is subject to other than medical criteria of evaluation: legal, political, religious, and aesthetic.

When illness is construed as incompetence of function, especially in social role behavior, and health as competence, we are led directly to the issue of *positive* health. Many observers have argued that health is something quite different from the mere absence of conventional symptoms of illness, that it is in fact to be characterized by superior functioning. This is the burden, for example, of the World Health Organization's definition of health as "total physical, mental, and social well-being," rather than the absence of disease. Some concept of positive health seems to be essential to the effort of primary prevention—the fostering of good health, as contrasted to intervention in already-ill processes. Here we are really concerned with the attempt to strengthen individual and group capacity, to cultivate competent behavior. The idea of health as efficacy underlies most discussions of positive wellness, such as the excellent summary by Marie Jahoda in her *Current Concepts of Positive Mental Health*.[4] Professor Jahoda erects certain "inner" criteria (self-acceptance, self-mastery) and certain "outer" indices (realistic posture in interpersonal relations). The stress is on a general cognitive and emotional competence, a capacity for balancing the heart's desire with the way of the world.

We come at length to recognize that health and illness probably cannot be rigorously defined in a manner that will be appropriate to all people, places, and times. They are processes, even if we often speak in shorthand about "states of health." Their definition is the consequence of a series of social actions, combining inner judgments (self-perception) and outer evaluations (the observations of significant other people). Individuals vary both

[4] Marie Jahoda, *Current Concepts of Positive Mental Health*, Joint Commission on Mental Illness and Health, Monograph Series 1 (New York: Basic Books, 1958).

in their fulfillment of the diverse components of healthy functioning and in their exposure to situational demands upon behavior. As there are many kinds of "dis-ease," so there are many conceptions of health. The idea of health as functional competence in enacting social roles, however, steers us away from a flabby relativism. Although there are many models of healthy behavior, clearly shaped by different cultural and social milieux, the nature of human interaction sets important limits on what shall be judged healthy. The eminent anthropologist Clyde Kluckhohn pointed out, for example, that there are no societies in which entire uncommunicativeness (muteness) or random aggression are considered healthy or indeed acceptable behaviors. The *search* for definition is a vital activity, even if we foresee no final or fixed agreement. Out of the search, out of the provisional definitions that change with changing knowledge and with alterations of the social scene, is sure to evolve a fuller conception of man, a more ample way of thinking about what it means to be human. Defining health and illness is no parochial task, and it is far from a purely theoretical exercise. What we demand as health and deprecate as disease influences our inquiries, our care, and our total sweep of social medical action.

CHAPTER 2

Patient-Practitioner Relations[1]

In every medical action there are always two parties involved, the physician and the patient, or in a broader sense, the medical corps and society. Medicine is nothing else than the manifold relations between these two groups. The history of medicine, therefore, cannot limit itself to the history of the science, institutions, and characters of medicine, but must include the history of the patient in society, that of the physician, and the history of the relations between physician and patient.

HENRY E. SIGERIST [2]

Sigerist's assertion that health care is essentially a social relationship deserves special emphasis today because our era is distinguished by its focus on the technology of medicine. In the dense web of machinery, technique, testing, and computer processing that enfolds modern medicine, it is often easy to forget that the nub of the health system is found in the interplay between helper and helped. Patient-practitioner relationships are best viewed in the framework of social roles, of the attitudes and activities the two parties bring to the situation of care. This interaction of two or more persons, centering around the health needs of a single individual, is far from being a spontaneous hap-

---

[1] This chapter draws heavily on Robert N. Wilson, "Patient-Practitioner Relationships," in Howard Freeman, Sol Levine, and Leo Reeder (eds.), *The Handbook of Medical Sociology* (Englewood Cliffs, N.J.: Prentice-Hall, 1963).

[2] Henry E. Sigerist, in Felix Marti-Ibanez (ed.), *Henry E. Sigerist on the History of Medicine* (New York: M.D. Publications, 1960), p. 26.

pening. It is, rather, a more or less well-rehearsed confrontation in which the key participants have learned to expect certain things and to act in certain ways. Just as health and illness are subject to various definitions, so the pattern of activities designed to intervene in ill processes is phrased in different ways—and is always a social definition.

What is the implication of construing health care as a social role relationship? It means, first, that this interaction between a helping agent and a person needing help is patterned and, hence, shows predictable regularities. Sickness and health are too important in human affairs to be left to improvised chance encounters; rather, they are treated in ways that form part of man's culture, that have been passed among individuals as a social heritage.

If patient-practitioner relations are a patterned sector of culture, then they must be transmitted from those who know about them to those who do not. These roles are learned sequences of behavior. One of the prime difficulties in helping relationships, almost a leitmotif in modern medicine and public health, is that the parties to the transaction often do not learn the same things in the same ways. Thus, when they confront one another, they manifest attitudes and actions that are inappropriate to the other's perception of the health care situation. A great deal of helping takes place between people whose relationship is marked, at least initially, by formidable barriers to communication and mutual satisfaction. Within a given society, say the United States, the barriers may consist of differences in health sophistication (the physician is a professional, whereas the patient is an amateur, despite the occasional "professional" hypochondriac), differences in social status, and differences in racial or ethnic group membership. Between societies, as in the thrust to introduce Western medicine into the developing countries, all these barriers are compounded by divergent cultural milieux that may promote radically different assumptions about the nature of illness and about who should treat whom.

The concept of social role entails a basic mutuality, a meshing of viewpoints and activities. Each of the persons entering upon a role transaction must be familiar with both his own and the other's expectations and both his own and the other's probable sequence of behaviors. Because effective role behavior involves this degree of orientation, the patient-practitioner relationship demands considerable sophistication if the therapeutic yield is to be large.

It is apparent that neither of the parties can define his own role independently of his role partner. The helping agent's view of himself does not make up all of his role; the full meaning of acting as doctor or nurse rests also on the patient's conception of what a doctor or nurse is. Similarly, the role of the patient is composed both of subjective models of patienthood and of the helper's notions about what constitutes a good—or a bad—client.

The Asymmetry of Therapeutic Relations

We have asserted that the roles of treater and client must in important respects be mutually understood and mutually rewarding. However, this does not at all mean that practitioners and patients are equals in the therapeutic situation. In the nature of the case, some significant change is to be promoted in the behavior, the total state of health, of the patient. As the skilled person meets the unskilled and tries to alter the latter, the parties can no more be equals than are parent and child or teacher and student. The helping agent must have leverage to induce change. This leverage is generated by overall circumstances, notably the *professional prestige* and *situational authority* of the health agent and the *situational dependency* of the patient.

Health professionals, especially the physician, tend to rank fairly high in the prestige hierarchies of industrial societies, although this is much more true of the West than of, for example, the Soviet Union. But what is at issue in the therapeutic relationship is not the aura of high status; rather, it is the specific technical qualification of the healer, which lends him a position of power rooted in his having what the patient wants and needs. Thus even the ward attendant in a psychiatric hospital, whose general rank in society may be considerably lower than that of most of his patients, is, in the ward situation, endowed with a profound control over resources of reward and punishment.

The patient in many, if not most, health-care interactions assumes a passively dependent posture, for several reasons. The very existence of the relationship is premised on his being "out of his field," on not knowing what the treater knows. Further, the expert in any delivery of services has a certain initiative: even a shoeshine boy tells his customer how to place his feet. Much more important, however, is the vulnerable social and psychological stance of an individual who has defined himself or who has come to be defined by others as ill. Any brand of "dis-ease," from traumatic bodily injury to psychoneurosis, appears to foster a regression in the patient, a reversion in some degree to the role of dependent child. Some properties of being ill threaten the integrity of the person. He who adopts the sick role, for whatever reason, feels himself at least temporarily less than whole, weakened, open to the incursion of fear and trembling.

Physical illness threatens to strip off the veneer of civilization, rendering the person more animal, frail, and childlike. If severe, of course, it carries the realization of that final fear of death itself, of nonbeing. Mental illness renders the individual unsure, disoriented. As the sufferer is gauged incompetent and sees the incompetence mirrored in others' behavior toward him, he cannot but doubt himself. Again as the child, he requires the special reassurance of support and affection, of confirming evidence that he is worthy and that he really exists in a viable organization of selfhood.

Therapeutic relationships, then, are usually characterized by a pattern of imbalance in power, interest, and technical expertness. It is appropriate to inquire into the natural history of such relationships, beginning with the client's adoption of the sick role and pursuing the interaction through the course of treatment.

In Chapter 1, the process of definition in health and illness was rehearsed. We are aware that patients differ markedly in the speed with which they categorize themselves as sick and in the sorts of evidence they require to make such a determination. Once the sick role is assumed, however, it is shaped, at least in middle class American society, by the series of considerations set forth most clearly by Talcott Parsons:

1. This incapacity is intrepreted as beyond his powers to overcome by the process of decision-making alone; in this sense he cannot be "held responsible" for the incapacity. Some kind of "therapeutic" process, spontaneous or aided, is conceived to be necessary to recovery.

2. Incapacity defined as illness is interpreted as a legitimate basis for the *exemption* of the sick individual, to varying degrees, in varying ways, and for varying periods according to the nature of the illness, from his normal role and task obligations.
3. To be ill is thus to be in a partially and conditionally legitimated state. The essential condition of its legitimation, however, is the recognition by the sick person that to be ill is inherently undesirable, that he therefore has an obligation to "get well" and to cooperate with others to this end.
4. So far as spontaneous forces, the *vis medicatrix naturea,* cannot be expected to operate adequately and quickly, the sick person, and those with responsibility for his welfare, above all, members of his family, have an obligation to *seek competent help* and to cooperate with competent agencies in their attempts to help him get well; in our society, of course, principally medical agencies. The valuation of health, of course, also implies that it is an obligation to try to prevent threatened illness where this is possible.[3]

The first aspect of this model, the nonresponsibility of the patient and the idea that something more than an act of rational will is necessary to recovery, obviously paves the way to his entry upon a therapeutic course. His illness is not a condition he has brought wholly on himself, and he cannot be expected to repair it unhelped. Nonresponsibility fixes the ill person in a special variety of deviance from his society. Although he is unlike his fellows who are adjudged "well," he did not deliberately set himself apart. The exemption of the sick individual from "normal role and task obligations" is contingent upon his simultaneously striving toward an improved state of health. Here both the valuing of good health as a "good" and the enjoining to achieve a speedy bettering by the self-application of desire and energy are distinguishing features of certain patients in certain cultures—as in the middle class American variety. Whether or not the patient will indeed seek help and whether or not he determines the competence of that help by professional health standards are similarly qualified by his experience and social characteristics.

Interaction between treater and client is thus initially shaped by the client's assumption of the sick role, his seeking assistance.

[3] Talcott Parsons, *The Social System* (New York: Free Press, 1951), pp. 428–473.

It is clearly shaped as well by the practitioner's assumption of the helping role, by the technical and social psychological armamentarium that the professional brings to the encounter. A helping agent may be accurately viewed in several ways: knowledgeable teacher; confidant; skilled diagnostician or analyst; and "middleman" between pharmacological, surgical, or mechanical resources and the client. Basically, the helper's significance is perhaps best understood in his capacity as an agent of social control; he is one of society's representative figures in managing deviant behavior and sustaining social order. In this sense, the practitioner is conservative. He is engaged in restoring a measure of balance to the social system by enabling the ill person to resume his customary responsibilities and activities, that is, taking up again those social roles that have been reduced or cast into temporary abeyance as a condition of his entrance to the sick role.

One of Parsons' most penetrating insights into the sociology of medicine is his insistence that illness is indeed a form of deviance and that the energetic effort to bring the ill person back from the sick role to maximum social performance is as necessary to the environing society as it is desirable to the ill individual. The function of the helping relationship is thus not only (perhaps not even chiefly) to benefit the sufferer but also to benefit the society by restoring so far as possible a human resource who is contributory in getting necessary things done. Obviously, from the point of view of a social system as a network of relationships, illness signifies disruption and failure to enact the social roles on which the system rests—the familial, occupational, and other obligations carried by the well population. This is the real meaning of the definition of the sick role as temporary and undesirable. The doctor's office or the hospital room, for example, have somewhat the aura of sanctuary. But like the priest or lawyer, the physician offers only temporary respite, as a way station on the patient's path of reentry to normal social activity.

One of the most revealing angles of approach to therapy is the comparison of this relationship with that of parent and child, with the socialization process as elaborated most thoughtfully by Parsons. Socialization and therapy have interestingly similar characteristics as processes of social control, as asymmetrical relationships, as emotionally laden and directed toward a terminus in which the dependent party has become independent as a fully functioning member of his society. The emotional relearning of psychotherapy comes closer to the model of socialization than does general medical practice, but therapy of any sort is illumined by the comparison. Four major features of the relationship are singled out for analysis; these features have the activity of parent or therapist as their point of reference. They are: (1) Support, (2) Permissiveness, (3) Manipulation of reward, and (4) Denial of reciprocity. Briefly, they entail the following:

1. Support: the therapist expresses his obligation to be of assistance, to provide a stable figure on whom the patient may lean. He will be available, helpful, nurturant toward the patient's needs for dependency. It is understood, however, that the support is temporary and contingent on the patient's continuing efforts to get well.

2. Permissiveness: the therapist allows the patient to express feelings and indulge in actions which would not be acceptable in a nontherapeutic relationship. Again the dispensation is temporary and rooted in the idea that patient or child is for the moment unable to adhere strictly to ordinary norms of social intercourse. Permissiveness is granted with the justification that the patient, by reason of his illness, "can't help" doing certain things and cannot be held to usual expectations of responsibility.

3. Manipulation of reward: the therapist exerts leverage on the ill person by controlling certain rewards which are especially significant to the dependent party. As in child-rearing, the primary reward is probably approval, which can be offered or withheld at the discretion of the socializing or therapeutic agent. Rewards are given for doing the "right thing," for trying to "grow up" or to "get well."

4. Denial of reciprocity: the therapist, as a condition of the granting of support and permissiveness, withholds from the patient his own full interpersonal responsiveness. He keeps the relationship asymmetrical by refusing either to feel all the patient feels or to allow the patient access to his, the therapist's, true feelings. He will not meet fire with fire, irritation with irritation, adoration with adoration; for to do so

would be to sacrifice the independent terrain on which he stands, and with it the potential for helping the other.[4]

Assuredly the patient and child are not the same thing. One departs from a disturbed maturity, whereas the other is, by definition, immature. Doctor and parent are unlike in the magnitude of their involvement with the dependent party, the depth of their emotional linkage, and the range of their concerns for the other. Yet the processes of inducting an individual into society and of returning him to a full and sanctioned functioning in society are remarkably parallel. In particular, the patient's being as a child seems to be inseparable from the physical and emotional insult of illness, and the physician's being as a parent seems intrinsically commensurate with his superior knowledge and experience in the domain of health.

The sanctity of body and mind are matters too important to be submitted to an utterly rational calculus of anticipation and behavior. Doctor and patient are entrapped in the mysteries of life and their intercourse partakes of a religious flavor: no patient in extremity of suffering and anxiety can regard the physician as of like substance with himself; the curative path and the curative agent are necessarily endowed with transcendent qualities and approached with ardent faith rather than cool resolve. There are at least two salient sets of reasons why the doctor-patient relationship is pervaded by mystical-religious elements. The first involves the peculiar dependence of patient on physician, the giving over by one individual to another of critical decisions affecting not only the course of life but also in some instances the possibility of survival. In order for this extraordinary transaction to occur, the patient must view his doctor in a manner far removed from the prosaic and the mundane. He thus more or less consciously regards him as the possessor of charismatic qualities, of a magnetic and profound gift for leadership in affairs of health. There is, of course, a very great distance between the faith invested in a Navaho singer or a Caribbean spiritualist and the faith invested in a clinician at a university medical center. Yet every healing relationship contains a substratum of nonra-

[4] Talcott Parsons and Reneé Fox, "Illness, Therapy, and the Modern Urban Family," *Journal of Social Issues,* 8 (1952), 31–44.

tional awe, and every healer is endowed with at least a minimum of magical attributes.

A second root of the mystical and the religious lies in the character of medicine itself. Although the scope of phenomena that are amenable to empirical explanation and control in medicine has steadily been enlarged, especially during the first half of the twentieth century, the plethora of unanswered and presently unanswerable questions generates precisely the kind of basic uncertainty that underlies the religious impulse. Art and religion both attempt to hint at the ineffable and to bring pattern into the inexplicable flux of existence. Medicine remains an art-science, and one must be dubious about the proposition that clinical intuition will give way entirely to electronic computation of syndromes. The increasing relevance of psychotherapy to medicine in general, and perhaps particularly to the run of chronic ailments probably means that the domain of the incompletely formulated, the spontaneous, and the intuitive will remain large and may in some instances even expand.

We have, then, rehearsed certain features of the therapeutic interaction: definition of the person as ill; assumption of the sick role; and the treater's application of social control in levering illness toward wellness. Perhaps the very asymmetry of these patterns, together with the ambiguities inherent in treating when health knowledge is inexact, contributes to a final feature of the helping relationship, namely its frequent lack of agreed upon closure. One might contend that enhancing an individual's state of health is literally an endless operation. A health state can presumably always be improved, especially in cases like the chronic and mental ills, where the criteria of evaluation are so murky. Just as the child-rearing model permits of no easy, convenient terminus—When, if ever, is an individual to be judged finally "adult" or "socialized"?—so the therapeutic model is laden with an uncertainty of conclusion. The health professional is evidently best equipped on technical grounds to announce that treatment has run its course, that all has been done that can be done. Yet the patient has an initiative in maintaining or breaking off the relationship. Sigmund Freud, of course, posed the question for psychotherapy in 1937 in his "Analysis Terminable and Interminable," but today with the rise of chronicity and increasing public health efforts to monitor and sustain the health of large groups, the issue of termination may become still more important to medicine at large. It may in fact become necessary to redefine patient-practitioner relations as intermittent and lifelong, after the fashion implied in the nostalgic image of the nineteenth-century country doctor, rather than as relations marked by sharp beginnings and endings.

The Ideal of Asymmetry: Some Reservations

Of course, the model of professional leverage and cooperative patienthood sketched above is just that: a model often approached in the conventional doctor-patient interaction of private medical practice in this country, but one that is inadequate to the complexities of today's multiple health enterprises. There are at least three sets of grave reservations about this model; they involve *the nature of the illness, the characteristics of those to be helped,* and *the numbers and kinds of treaters active in health care.*

The features of the sick role set forth by Parsons apply readily to acute illness, to those health states the patient can easily recognize and can have some confidence in surmounting with the practitioner's help. Subtle or chronic disability, however, is quite another matter. An individual with a socially "acceptable" neurotic style may not seek help, may even actively avoid help, and yet exert a deleterious effect on others' lives and fall far short of competencies and enjoyments he might potentially grasp. A paraplegic, or in a less severe example, a patient with chronic joint or organic disease, can scarcely expect to "get well" in the terms suggested by the sick role model, however willing he is to collaborate with helping agents. Rather, the practitioner is intent on partial restoration of the patient's ability to cope with social role demands and on an educative process designed to help him live with his disease.

Furthermore, the asymmetrical pattern of conventional helping relationships is modified if the client is a target of preventive, rather than strictly therapeutic, maneuvers. A vast range of contemporary health work is concerned not with restoring a single patient from the sick role to normal functioning but with maintaining and improving the state of health of large populations. Patient-practitioner relations must of course be different when the "patient" is a population group or an entire community and when the condition to be treated is not a frankly disabling illness but, for example, smoking behavior or local water pollution. The nature of the "illness" in such instances implies that the health agent be persuasive rather than authoritative and that possibilities of change hinge much more crucially on self-determined shifts in individual and collective behavior.

Those to be helped by modern medicine do not necessarily come to a practitioner as active seekers of care. Far more often, particularly in public health, the agent of care lacks the leverage inherent in his being asked for his aid. Instead, he must persuade the potential client that certain actions (being screened for tuberculosis or cancer, for example) are desirable or that changes in his behavior would be of value outweighing the pleasures of indulgence or inertia. Colloquially posed, the question frequently is: How do you get people to want what's good for them? How, that is, does one convince a target population that what a health professional deems worthy is in fact so desirable for them that health benefits will exceed the costs?

The ideal therapeutic pattern is based on a traditional one-to-one interaction between doctor and patient. We have pointed out that the patient today may often be a population rather than a sick individual. Similarly, the practitioner is less and less commonly a solo agent providing comprehensive aid; instead, a coordinated team of health professionals is engaged in a joint approach to medical risks. This inevitably means that the pattern of "resocialization" in the classic doctor-patient framework cannot occur on the same terms. To emphasize only a single difference, the client being helped by a battery of professionals can hardly muster the intensity of trust (and dependency) that undergirds the growth of transference in a psychotherapeutic encounter between *a* patient and *a* physician. The thoroughgoing identification of treated with treater implied in the concept of transference must clearly be diluted and redistributed, or at length, other social psychological mechanisms must be cultivated and brought into play.

Class Barriers to Communication

If the health professional and the patient differ in their mastery of health knowledge and techniques, this basic imbalance may be exaggerated by other dissimilarities in the social worlds from which they come. And, indeed, the gulf in technical vocabulary and in the conceptual framework through which illness is viewed tends to widen as the social class origins of the two parties become more remote from one another. To a very considerable extent, the ideal taking of the sick role reflects a middle class value pattern on which physician and client agree. This pattern emphasizes the merits of individual responsibility, deliberate striving and grooming of the self toward health, and mastery and activism in the carrying out of normal social roles, particularly in the occupational sphere. Above all, the pattern assumes that rational problem solving is the only viable behavior in the face of difficulty. Health is to be sought and illness to be expeditiously cured; the fate of misfortune is not to be passively bemoaned or stoically accepted.

Yet, of course, the motivations and expectations that underlie this posture can be taken for granted only in a slice of the population. This slice is the advantaged, privileged sector of our society, overwhelmingly white, educated, and affluent. Patients are well-fed and well-clothed, comfortably housed, and steadily employed. If the world is not quite everywhere and always their oyster, it is at any rate a social universe to be mastered, manipulated, controlled in the interest of attaining the prestige and possessions that advertisers knowingly term "the good things of life." What of the large numbers of Americans who lie outside this advantaged sector but who exhibit an abundance of health needs?

A good deal of evidence, discussed more fully in Chapter 8, indicates that individuals of lower socioeconomic status not only have a greater chance of contracting the majority of illnesses but are also least likely to seek and receive adequate health care. Beyond the strictly economic aspects of the situation (and these are still not at all negligible, despite the movement toward a more solid flooring of services for the poor), we find a whole complex of motivational and life-style features that render patient-practitioner relations uneasy. Helper and helped do not speak the same language, but this is not merely a question of technical vocabulary.

To be sure, research shows that the poor and members of some minority ethnic groups misunderstand a major fraction of the terms conventionally used by doctors and nurses.[5] Probably more important, however, are differences in the assumptions that lie behind the words. To take but a single example, a distinctive concept of time and its meaning is implicit in the traditional medical helping arrangement. This concept assumes that people are highly aware of the passage of time and that they monitor time as a normal aspect of their behavior. Such awareness is clearly essential to self-medication and the keeping of medical appointments. Further, it assumes a specific orientation toward future time in which people build toward a desirable state of affairs in which, for instance, they exercise for progressive reattainment of muscle function or look forward to completing a course of unpleasant or inconvenient medication. But this view represents a middle class orientation to the clock and the calendar; millions of lower class patients do not habitually monitor time, living instead by sun, season, and the fabric of significant life events.[6] Millions, too, as described by Allison Davis,[7] do not defer present pleasures or schedule themselves in favor of a desired future. Their lives have not taught them that a concept of the future is workable, because in their experience of hazardous daily living the future has never arrived, the rewards for this sort of husbanding of self and resources have not been received.

Instances of such divergence in orientation could be multiplied. In psychotherapy it has commonly been found that many lower class patients lack habits of self-expression and introspection and are simply not used to objectifying the emotional life. In many helping relationships, the avenues of discussion and flow of information are clogged by the disadvantaged patient's often

[5] Julian Samora, Lyle Saunders, and Richard F. Larson, "Medical Vocabulary Knowledge Among Hospital Patients," *Journal of Health and Human Behavior,* 2 (Summer 1961), 83–92.

[6] John Horton, "Time and Cool People," *Trans-action,* (April 1967), pp. 5–12.

[7] Allison Davis, "The Motivation of the Underprivileged Worker," in William Foote Whyte (ed.), *Industry and Society* (New York: McGraw-Hill, 1946), pp. 84–106.

well-founded mistrust and fear of authority figures. His evasive or mutely accepting posture does not augur well for a sustained therapeutic interchange.

And, to be sure, conversations between the classes are not thwarted solely by obdurate or unaware behavior on the part of lower class clients. The health professional wears his own perceptual blinders. Not only may he be limited to a middle class stereotype of the responsive and responsible patient and yearn for the client to be more nearly like himself, but he also customarily carries a certain moral freight. The message on this freight is that the disadvantaged patient is not just different but morally bad or inferior. The pattern of illness itself may be unconsciously interpreted as a tangible sign of the lack of grace: if the patient had cared for himself and ordered his life differently, perhaps his health state would be better.

Patient-practitioner relations between individuals of widely varying social class identities are therefore colored by a series of difficulties. Some may be overcome by shrewd and persistent education of *both* the health professional and his prospective client, by education to make them more aware of one another. Some may be mitigated through the employment of new varieties of health worker; for example, there is increasing effort to train auxiliary personnel as a species of health intermediary who can stand between the classes and interpret in both directions. Perhaps most critical, however, will be attempts to discover or invent new models of the relationship itself, to find effective alternatives to the classic model of therapeutic asymmetry. Such alternatives may involve changes in the number and kind of helping roles, as in the case of the health intermediary. They are also likely to entail a concentration on preventive, as well as therapeutic, health care. Above all, fresh models of the interplay between patient and practitioner will be guided by principles of continuous and comprehensive care in contrast to the urgent intervention traditionally applied at the stage of frank disorder. The relation of helper to helped will be less time-bound and place-bound and more realistically attuned to the individual's total life history.

Cultural Differences

An important share of American medicine's activities is directed to the health care of patients whose culture differs markedly from the prevailing culture of the United States. Part of the process of development in the "developing" nations is a health process. This must be the case, both because industrial productivity demands a population functioning at high levels of wellness and because westernization itself generates health risks as a fraction of the human price to be paid for rapid change. There no longer seems to be any point in debating the desirability of the great tide of change from traditional agricultural societies to urban industrial ones. The change is in fact desired by those who must change, and no romantic nostalgia for a less hurried and harried way of life appears to stand a chance when stacked against automobiles, refrigerators, and the civility of the city. This is not to say, of course, that modernization is necessarily a quick or easy process; it is simply to reaffirm that industrialization is overwhelmingly the *direction* of development in the disadvantaged two-thirds of the world.

The basic consideration in the introduction of Western scientific medicine to non-Western cultures is that the health techniques and knowledge cannot be transferred as isolated parcels. That is, Western models of medical practice or of health theory do not stand alone as cultural fragments but are woven into a larger system of custom and value. Patient-practitioner relations represent peculiarly interesting and complicated conversations across cultures. Lyle Saunders has provided perhaps the clearest and most comprehensive statements of what cultural differences mean for the social role of the practitioner. He said:

> When the practice of medicine involves the application of elements of the institution of medicine in one culture to the people of another, or from one subculture to members of another subculture within the same cultural group, what is done or attempted by those in the healing roles may not be fully understood or correctly evaluated by those in the patient roles. Conversely, the responses of those on the patient side of the interaction may not conform to the expectations of those on the healing side. To the extent that this

occurs, the relationship may be unsatisfactory to everyone concerned.

When persons of widely dissimilar cultural or subcultural orientations are brought together in a therapeutic relationship, the probability of a mutually satisfactory outcome may be increased if those in the healing roles know something of their own culture and that of the patient and are aware of the extent to which behavior on both sides of the relationship is influenced by cultural factors. An even higher probability of satisfaction may result if the professional people are willing and able to modify elements from their medicine so as to make them fit the expectations of the laymen with whom they are working.[8]

The hazards we mentioned concerning the health care of the lower class patient by a middle class professional are repeated and magnified in cross-cultural medicine. Once again, the helping agent is called on to examine his own unstated assumptions about the "proper" roles of the parties to the transaction, to strip out the necessary therapeutic aspects of the relationship from the merely conventional features. Health professionals in foreign settings must, as Saunders avers, look closely at their own culture and attempt an empathic reaching out toward an understanding of the patient's culture. Above all, they must be sensitive to the fact that a given item of health behavior is part of a system that transcends health affairs as such; not only does this systematic character shape the meaning of health events, but it also implies that health changes will influence, and be influenced by, other sorts of social change.

Examples of patient-practitioner relations going wrong in cross-cultural interaction are legion, and as one might expect, examples of successful health care are far fewer. One of the familiar difficulties for the male physician is the reluctance of women in many traditional cultures to be examined and treated if this involves intimate access to the body. Another prominent sequence of misunderstanding occurs when the Western health agent underestimates the relevance of kinship ties to patient behavior. He may regard the patient's relatives as rank intruders if they accompany the patient to his office or insist on being always present on home visits. Yet in many societies the illness of one

[8] Lyle Saunders, *Cultural Difference and Medical Care* (New York: Russell Sage Foundation, 1954), p. 8.

member is a profoundly family affair, in which relatives lend strength, rather than disrupt therapy, through their presence.

Once again, as in the cross-social class situation, effective helping can often be achieved by utilizing health intermediaries who stand between Western medical professionals and an indigenous population. The creation of new auxiliary health roles of this kind has proved to be of value in several settings. A notable example is the Cornell Many Farms project in which a Navaho intermediary, termed a "health visitor," served in a tuberculosis treatment program as go-between for Western practitioners in the clinic and Navaho patients in their widely scattered homes.

Staging Therapeutic Dramas

As Erving Goffman has brilliantly argued,[9] all social relationships are governed in part by the physical settings in which they occur. The stages where therapeutic processes are acted out vary and with them the whole social psychological tone of the encounter. In modern medical practice in the United States, for instance, the prototypical stage is the physician's private office. This is where Parsons' versions of sick role and asymmetrical relations, as well as the classic maneuvers of psychotherapy, come, if ever, to full flower. In the office the practitioner has maximum control over the terms of the relationship: he can arrange timing, furnishings, and the roles of assisting personnel to suit himself and to impress the client in the manner desired.

A quite different pattern may emerge when the setting shifts to the hospital or clinic or to the patient's household. In the hospital many more people are involved in treatment. Their influence is as direct as the aide's taking a blood sample and as indirect as the housekeeping worker's heightening morale through a sunny greeting or gestures that suggest genuine care. In any event, the locus of therapy is diffused, and the physician is himself subject to a variety of organizational constraints. He thus cannot exert the same kind of leverage on the patient's total behavior. On the other hand, of course, the patient is likely to be

[9] Erving Goffman, *The Presentation of Self in Everyday Life* (Edinburgh: University of Edinburgh Social Science Research Center, 1958).

still more passive in the hospital situation. He is stripped of his identity along with his clothes and literally at the whim of those who attend him.

In the household, presumably, the distribution of initiatives and powers is again rearranged. Here the patient and his family can much more nearly guide the stream of interaction. If future patterns of care, as seems very likely, involve a renewed emphasis on home care, therapeutic styles may undergo significant revision.

Even further removed from the one-to-one isolated relationship in the doctor's office are the growing efforts at prevention and early treatment that take place in "natural" community settings. A rudimentary helping relationship may be staged at the occupational setting, for example, or at the school. Such interactions commonly involve helping agents other than health professionals; these agents may provide direct early care in consultation with a health expert. In some schools today, for instance, teachers are coming to serve as "treaters" of children's mental health problems. The remarkable experimental program at Woodlawn, a low income Negro section of Chicago, seems to indicate that the emotional health of the young child may be fostered by the efforts of teachers and classmates to cope with aberrant behavior through group discussion and illustration. In this setting the health professional, the psychiatrist, stays well in the background; his role is that of consultant and planner rather than that of primary therapist.

Helping relationships in the future are unlikely to be confined to the therapeutic arenas—the physician's office or hospital bedside—in which the helper can stage-manage and manipulate at will. If the settings shift, the relationships will also shift. Different physical and social spaces will demand that the preventive or healing interaction be modulated, probably in the direction of a more nearly symmetrical pattern, a discourse composed between equals.

Toward New Therapeutic Patterns

This discussion has systematically distorted the nature of contemporary medical practice by its enforced concentration on a single model of doctor-patient relations. It has focused on the therapeutic pairing that consists of the independent medical professional vis-à-vis one patient, whether it be in the context of general medicine or of psychotherapy. Today, many other models are in effect, and one may discern a variety of future alternatives.

The most pronounced shift in the traditional Western therapeutic dyad is probably a departure from the dyad itself. Increasingly, the patient is involved not in an isolated two-person social system but in a medical team effort in which the physician is first among equals rather than unique healer. A paramount issue of the future may be the redefinition of the doctor's role as a collaborative one and the patterning of team medicine for maximum therapeutic efficacy. The future of medical practice will probably rest on a detailed meshing of medicine, nursing, social work, administration, and perhaps even social science.

Complementing the apparent breakup of the exclusive one-to-one relationship from the practitioner's side, there is a growing disposition to involve other family members and significant figures in the patient's life space. Although this disposition is, of course, most obvious in psychotherapy, following the lead of child-guidance clinics that treat families rather than disturbed children, it is also relevant to general practice.

Michael Balint, Iago Galdston, James Halliday, and others are now beginning to discern a model of social medicine in which the practitioners, with the help of auxiliary specialists, try to unite psychological, social, and biological orientations in therapy. They envision a patient-practitioner relationship that will monitor the patient's ill and healthy life course rather than limit itself to the treatment of specific disease entities.

The comprehensive medical care of the future seems certain to engender new helping agents, new concepts of therapy, and new settings of care. A concerted push by public and private agencies, spurred by recent federal health legislation, is leading toward a more rationally planned system of medical services. Fresh schemes of care will emphasize area-wide health planning designed to achieve coordination of myriad health facilities. The patient—the focus of these efforts—will, it is hoped, come to enjoy a better coordinated array of services and a more nearly continuous history of preventive and curative encounters. Candor and accuracy force us to confess that we cannot now envision with perfect confidence what the future of patient-practitioner relations will be. What *does* appear sure is that there will be important changes in the patterns of helping that will accompany other major changes in our society. The interpersonal flow between treater and treated will become a more visible public concern and will be increasingly exposed to scrutiny by the society at large.

CHAPTER 3

Health Professions

Medicine is one of the dominant fields of activity in American society. The care of a population that now numbers over 200 million and that is demanding ever-higher standards of service requires a very large labor force of health workers. In sheer economic terms, health ranks among the largest of United States "industries." And in the more general framework of values, health is widely cherished as a basic right, to be legitimately possessed by the citizens of an affluent country. Those who practice what is so desired, who have technical mastery of the possibility for achieving a state of good health, are inevitably important figures.

First in importance, by tradition, prestige, income, and the deference of popular opinion, is the physician. Doctors are very highly rated by the public in all surveys of who's who in American society. This stature is buttressed by the physician's technical knowledge and skill and by his formally defined authority in the domain of health. Underlying the doctor's commanding social role are the basic psychological factors rehearsed earlier: the patient's dependency, the necessary awe with which the sufferer regards the healer, and the magical and religious properties constituting the doctor's charisma or magnetic attractiveness.

Affairs were not always thus. The history of medicine offers convincing evidence of rise and fall in the physician's stock. In the France of Louis XIV, for example, even the most eminent physicians were regarded as rather clever and lofty servants. The head of the Paris medical faculty usually received a tip under his plate when he dined out with members of the nobility. Physicians distrusted one another in public, and the faculties of rival medical schools openly termed their competitors charlatans or worse. Medicine as a discipline in seventeenth-century France still clung to the dicta set forth by Galen: the science was philosophical and disputatious, not observational or experimental. There was comparatively little any doctor could do for his patient beyond the rituals of purging and bleeding, techniques that were applied with enthusiasm to already weakened patients. The barber-surgeons inspired very little confidence in surgical intervention. All in all, it was probably not too unjust to suggest, as one contemporary writer did, that Louis survived to the age of seventy-seven despite the efforts of his physicians. It is well to remember, when considering the relatively modest historical estate of the doctor, that only in the early twentieth century did patients consulting a medical professional come to have better than an even chance of being helped by his ministrations.

Because his role has a very long history and because he now undergoes a much more rigorous education than any other health professional, the physician is the model for the host of newer health professions. In a sense, each variety of health worker gauges his status and professional selfhood in terms of how closely he approaches the doctor on a scale of privilege and responsibility. The physician shares with the hospital a fundamental legal responsibility for what happens to the patient. This very real and serious obligation, one that is frequently made active by the increasing possibility of malpractice suits, is complemented by the doctor's traditional position as leader of the health care team. Each professional role that grows out of the enormous variety and complexity of modern medicine tends to be patterned on the ideal image of the physician, with his technical mastery and basic independence of action. The doctor-as-model serves the positive goal of encouraging high aspirations and standards of practice on the part of other health workers. On the other hand, his exalted status is in some respects an inflated, unrealistic aim for most of the auxiliary professions. They cannot, by definition, achieve entire parity with him, and their efforts to come close often entail frustration and damage both pride and performance.

The Nature of the Professional

In professional settings, as distinct from most other work settings in our society, the aspiring worker can hope to rise in status and income only within his own professional cadre. That is, the nurse or laboratory technician cannot expect to attain the position of the M.D. by superior job performance; a health worker must go "outside" the work situation and pursue specialized education in order to rise higher than the top of his own occupational tree. Hence, we have the classic picture of "blocked mobility" that plagues hospitals and other health organizations. The vexed questions surrounding the relationship of the medical profession to the other health professions are in the process of constant reexamination. Two paths of change are currently visible: the revision of at least certain physicians' roles to a more nearly colleaguelike, or first among equals, pattern; and the clearer definition of ancillary health roles to provide specific rewards and distinctions in a channel partially separate from the physician-dominated hierarchy.

Our notions of the "professional" are simultaneously rooted in the history of occupations in our culture and subject to change as the tempos and styles of work itself change. In traditional usage the professions are those occupations adhering to ancient patterns of special learnedness and altruism, as exemplified in the ideal image of the priest or lawyer. This history leads to the designation of work roles as more or less professional, depending upon how closely they hew to a set of criteria, such as those advanced by Ernest Greenwood. They are:

1. A system of theoretical knowledge which serves as the basis for the professional skill.
2. Professional authority: the power to prescribe a course of action for a client because of superior knowledge, for example, doctor's orders.
3. Approval of authority claims by the community.
4. A code of ethics designed to protect the client, provide service

to the community, and provide a basis for elimination of un-
ethical practitioners.

5. Professional culture patterns consisting of values (for example,
the conviction that the professional service is valuable to the
community), norms which provide guides for behavior in
professional practice, symbols of professional status such as
the title "Doctor" and the concept of a professional career.[1]

Clearly, the physician fits this cloth well, as is seen in Greenwood's recurrent use of him as exemplar. Other health professionals just as clearly partake of several elements in the description, although usually in a less thoroughgoing fashion than does
the doctor. The nurse is most nearly comparable on several items;
however, neither her theoretical knowledge nor her authority
(and accompanying community acceptance of her claim to expertness) matches the physician's. Among other allied professionals who approximate doctor and nurse rather closely are such
figures as the hospital administrator, the social worker, and the
behavioral scientist. On the other hand, numerous groups of
health workers crave the appellation "professional," despite their
involvement in an occupational milieu that is quite distant from
these traditional criteria.

Changing styles of work and the attempt to win the title of
profession for its honorific overtones are leading steadily toward
professionalization of health occupations. Howard S. Becker asserts that it may be sensible to jettison the conventional concept,
to:

Take a radically sociological view, regarding professions simply as
those occupations which have been fortunate enough in the politics
of today's work world to gain and maintain possession of that
honorific title. On this view, there is no such thing as the "true"
profession, and no set of characteristics necessarily associated with
the title. There are only those work groups which are commonly
regarded as professions and those which are not.

Such a definition takes as central the fact that "profession" is an
honorific title, a term of approbation. It recognizes that profession
is a collective symbol and one that is highly valued. It insists that

[1] Ernest Greenwood, "Attributes of a Profession," in S. Nosow and
W. F. Form (eds.), *Man, Work, and Society* (New York: Basic
Books, 1962), p. 207.

"profession" is not a neutral and scientific concept but, rather, . . . a *folk concept*, a part of the apparatus of the society we study, to be studied by knowing how it is used and what role it plays in the operations of that society.[2]

Whatever definition of the professions we adopt, workers in the health fields are eager to merit the honor of such a self-image —and not merely honor, of course, but also the whole train of perquisites and responsibilities that attach themselves to established fields like medicine. One of the most striking aspects of contemporary medicine, indeed, is the exquisite specialization of skills that has been associated with the explosion of scientific health knowledge and techniques. This specialization, in turn, has spurred a desire on the part of each work group to render its own province of activity both distinctive and meritorious. We find, then, a sustained battle among specialists for a favored place in the professional sun. In the process each health specialty strives to take unto itself the sorts of characteristics summarized by Greenwood. Thus each is careful to claim a distinctive body of knowledge and skill that is clearly distinguished from neighboring specialties; each is proud of its historical development (however brief that development may have been); each embraces a strictly phrased ethical code; and each tries to mount a rigorous requirement of training for aspirants and to burnish a public image that will accurately reflect its cherished capabilities.

Two primary influences are at work in expanding the types and sheer numbers of health professionals. The first is the subdivision of the health task into ever more precise and limited components. The often satirized pattern of galloping specialization is probably an inevitable consequence of complexity and accumulation of knowledge. The second influence is the thrust toward a far more comprehensive notion of what health care entails, linked to a growing population and a growing conviction that health services should be available to all who need them. The thrust toward a more global definition of adequacy in care stems both from within the health professions, as leaders recognize the per-

[2] Howard S. Becker, "The Nature of a Profession," in Nelson B. Henry (ed.), *Education for the Professions* (Chicago: University of Chicago Press, 1962), p. 32.

vasiveness of illness and the multiplicity of its causes, and from without, as the consuming public raises its expectations of health and lowers its tolerance for "dis-ease."

If the health task today is more complex and more nearly all-inclusive, giving rise to varieties of new specialists, this very trend toward a finer division of labor carries a built-in contradiction. That is, the quest for adequacy of health services, for knowing more about the patient and helping him more thoroughly, simultaneously fosters a theory of integration and a practice of fragmentation. Health theory, as well as daily observation, dictates a renewed attention to the "whole" patient—not only to the total biosocial psychological individual but also to the totality of his setting in family and community relationships. Yet the specialization of the health professions is in one sense divisive of the patient, and a key problem inheres in efforts to link specialists together, so that the patient's wholeness is affirmed in treatment.

The health professions may be seen to be enmeshed in a series of social role relationships, each of which is in important respects problematic. In Chapter 2 we analyzed certain features of the professional's role vis-à-vis the patient. In addition, the health worker enacts roles with his fellow professionals, with allied specialists, and with a variety of persons involved in the staffing of medical care organizations.

One of the hallmarks of a profession by almost any definition is that it is in significant respects a self-contained fraternity, a closed group of those who share common ideas, skills, and a posture toward experience. The degree of inwardness or esoteric sharing, and hence of exclusiveness, varies from occupation to occupation, but all health professions are marked by distinctive languages, duties, and a sense of craft that cannot be readily shared with those outside. A fraternal dedication and feeling of colleagueship has several implications. On the one hand, it usually means that strong bonds exist within the profession and that all members experience a heightened morale and a conviction of worthwhileness in their occupational identity. In addition, health professionals feel responsible for one another and much concerned to maintain a set of work standards that will bolster the profession's public image. On the other hand, this very dedication and "we-feeling" often creates difficulties in interprofessional relations: If the individual invests so much of himself in a pattern of occupational loyalty, can he then stretch his identity to embrace other health workers or the whole medical institution in which work occurs? Can the individual be dissuaded from considering himself first a physician, nurse, or physical therapist, and only second, a member of a therapeutic team or of a hospital-as-society?

Interprofessional Relations

Interprofessional relations are closely bound up with the newness (and hence, often, the insecurity) of the health professions, with their intense quest of prestige, and with the rapidly shifting definitions of work roles. How a member of a given profession will behave toward a member of another is colored by the sometimes brittle sense of honor held by the individual and by the relative prestige each profession currently enjoys. Above all, interprofessional collaboration, so essential to the patient's welfare, is subject to the flow of agreement and disagreement about each occupation's proper domain of work. An especially pertinent illustration of these matters may be seen in the nursing profession and in the nurse's relation to other health workers, notably to the doctor.

Historically, of course, the nursing role evolved as that of handmaiden to the physician. The nurse was to offer the afflicted a benevolent and continuous attention while she served the physician as a helping pair of hands and eyes that constituted an extension of his own energies. Her subordination to the doctor in all events was taken for granted because her role was explicitly couched as an auxiliary one and because, moreover, she was typically a female in occupational pairing with a culturally defined dominant male. Yet the steady professionalization of nursing in the hundred years since Florence Nightingale's "invention" of this occupation in the Crimean War has led to radical change in the nurse's status and duties, with greatly increased variety of participation in health care. Today, the nurse may be an administrator, a teacher, a research scientist, or a frontline therapist (as in the case of the public health nurse). She may have a level of education ranging from that of the licensed practical nurse to that of the Ph.D.

Within the profession there is constant debate centering around conceptions of what nursing "really" is, what might be the core of the role, and what style of training is appropriate to optimal performance in any of several medical settings. The nurse-administrator may be thought to have relinquished the salient part of her traditional role in bedside care, with tender attentiveness to patient needs being left by default to lesser trained auxiliaries. The technically proficient nurse-therapist may be viewed as encroaching on the physician's territory of treatment. A college educated nurse who has mastered advanced techniques in the health sciences may find herself relegated in practice to the ancient structure of subordination to the doctor. Thus we find a role in ferment, exposed to constant readjustment of professional self-image and of relationships to other health workers.

The general problem of role definition runs throughout the interactions among health professionals. Another vivid example is seen in the psychiatric treatment team. Here the participants are several in number, usually including at least the physician, nurse, psychologist, social worker, ward attendant, and often encompassing such other figures as the occupational therapist. In one sense, each member has the "same" job: to reeducate the patient toward ordered intrapsychic and interpersonal functioning. Yet each also possesses certain distinctive skills and has staked out a customary sphere of activity. They must develop a common language and a mode of working together for the patient's benefit. But harmonious relations are not easily attained because the psychiatric task is itself difficult and the various professionals tend to be at once competitors and collaborators. William A. Rushing's incisive conclusion from his study of a mental hospital staff may be cited:

> If this book does nothing else, however, we think it shows that once the problems of adequate financing and competent personnel have been solved, other problems appear. For once you gather under the same roof a number of different professional groups with overlapping skills, you may invite the problems of competition for prestige and salary, conflicting conceptions of role duties, desires —and demands—for greater autonomy and independence, and other problems which create conflict among personnel and add problems for the administrator. Only the naïve believe that once the problems of economics and personnel have been solved the

dedication and competence of mental health professionals will prevent the occurrence of organizational conflict and tension.[3]

Interprofessional relations will be in still greater turmoil during the next decade, as administrators experiment with novel patterns of organization and fresh techniques of care emerge. The demand for comprehensive, community-centered health care imposes an obligation on professionals to rethink the scope of their cherished domains and to seek more precise definitions of therapeutic tasks.

Intraprofessional Relations

Two avenues of insight into the nature of a profession are the study of education for the professional role and the study of internal professional structure. Each of these patterns—the training of recruits and the self-organization of the membership—reveals important strains and positive features of the professional role from the inside, reflecting its favored self-image as well as its self-doubts. Thus there have been many efforts to capture the essence of the medical profession by analyzing the student's career in medical school. Similarly, a profession's internal organization indicates how members believe they should conduct themselves and how they prefer to be represented to the larger society.

Professional education has been realistically seen to have a double focus: the technical preparation of an individual for competent performance in a health task and the less formal grooming of the neophyte in the values and styles of professional conduct. The intellectual base of theory and data and the work skills entailed in the health job are presented to students in an increasingly intensive and sophisticated form. Curricula reflect the changes in professional role definition, especially the expansion of roles to embrace more varieties of technical mastery. Educational experiment has had great vitality in the health fields as they search for superior teaching forms and try to prepare young people for a multitude of activities. In medicine, nursing, and other areas there have been notable innovations. In recent years these innovations have been particularly directed to bringing the

[3] William A. Rushing, *The Psychiatric Professions* (Chapel Hill: University of North Carolina Press, 1964), p. 259.

student into more intimate and realistic interaction with patients. The aspiring doctor, for example, is given earlier and more fully responsible involvement with a series of patients or a series of families, in the hope that he will gain a firm idea of comprehensive and continuous health care.

Much of the educational change in the health professions is being addressed to what many observers consider the most glaring defect in American medicine: the gulf between technical medical proficiency and the application of this proficiency to the health needs of the public. Our *capacity* to serve, in terms of knowledge and technique, seems to far outstrip our ability to *deliver* service at the points of greatest urgency. It might well be argued that the health professional of the future must become as adept in interpersonal relations as he may be in biology or chemistry; his knowledge of social structure must come more nearly to match his knowledge of cell structure.

That part of professional education that inculcates values and informally coaches the aspiring individual in the preferred behavior of the mature professional is less easy to observe than the formal curriculum. In analogy to the child's experience of growing up in a given society, the making of a professional has been described as "adult socialization." The young student is shaped by his superiors and his peers, as the child is shaped in the family, until he comes close to a professional model. Adult socialization directs our attention to all the subtle cues older professionals pass on to younger; it encompasses the tones of voice, the expression, the language of gesture, the import of things that are *not* said as well as things that are. The overall growth of the student hinges not merely on what is intentionally conveyed to him as information but equally importantly on the influence of established professionals who figure as the models—the ideal images —of his own future professional self. And if older professionals serve as exemplars, then fellow students also exert a potent force. Students learn from one another in several ways. Perhaps most crucially, they learn to be members of a special culture, a preprofessional group that foreshadows the later development of colleague relationships. The significance of tutelage in values as a part of professional education is underlined by Robert K. Merton:

The schools thus have the double function of transmitting to students the *cognitive* standards of knowledge and skill and the *moral* standards of values and norms. Both sets of standards are essential to the proficient practice of medicine.[4]

And again:

Since numerous kinds of pressures may be exerted upon private practitioners to depart from what they know to be the most appropriate kind of medical care, it becomes functionally imperative that they acquire, in medical school, those values and norms which will make them less vulnerable to such deviations. It is in this direct sociological sense that the acquisition of appropriate attitudes and values is as central as the acquisition of knowledge and skills to training for the provision of satisfactory medical care.[5]

Health professions are marked by a very interesting species of internal organization, one that underlines the independence of the profession from outside or lay authority, at the same time that it stresses the interdependence of individuals on one another. All professions aspire to be in significant respects self-regulating. This is partly based on the desire to exercise specialized judgments free from inappropriate restrictions—to a considerable extent only a peer can evaluate the work of a professional. Partly, too, self-policing is a badge of occupational status. The more highly ranked an occupation or an individual, the greater the scope of discretionary activity, of liberty to choose the ends and means of work. As we shall see in Chapter 4, the striking autonomy of the health professions in pursuit of medical goals is increasingly circumscribed today by the demands of efficiency in work flow and by newer conceptions of the public interest in health. The administrator in the hospital necessarily encroaches on certain traditional professional prerogatives as hospitals become more complexly scheduled. The "third-party" payer for medical care in like fashion inevitably intrudes to some degree on the internal professional evaluation of work procedures. Despite these strictures, relationships among colleagues continue to be

[4] Robert K. Merton, George G. Reader, and Patricia L. Kendall (eds.), *The Student-Physician* (Cambridge: Harvard University Press, 1957), p. 76.
[5] *Ibid.*, p. 78.

vital not only for control of quality in professional work and for an endless process of mutual education but also for the sense of refreshed morale that springs from acceptance and fellowship.

The Professional of the Future

The health professions embody the excitement of steady growth in knowledge and the fascination of being absorbed in work that so obviously counts, that promises to make a major difference in peoples' lives. At the same time, their rapid change means frustration for those whose training becomes quickly obsolete, those who find themselves the possessors of "trained incapacity"—or, in John Dewey's remarkable phrase, "fit for an unfit fitness." Learning must very clearly be lifelong; the health professional has acute need for a personal flexibility. Considering the strains in these helping professions, the technical and interpersonal challenges that distinguish the daily task, and the extraordinarily modest financial rewards available to all but the physician, professionals can only be sustained by that deep "faith in vocation" and thorough commitment that Stephen Spender observed in the artist. Only a profound engagement with the world of health could keep them at their jobs.

Perhaps the most interesting contemporary feature of the health professions and the one most indicative of their victories and failures in American life is the immense pressure for more workers. This pressure reflects triumphs of medical technique as well as national affluence. It also reflects the failure to attract capable people in sufficient numbers and to open clear paths of satisfying schooling and achievement. As a result of all these trends, combined with an exploding demand for services, the health professions are now in a position in which they cannot possibly supply all the competent helping their society requires. Thus the current imperative for health workers to educate and accept a variety of nonprofessionals as a condition of getting their job done. If the United States is indeed becoming a "helping society," as many would contend, veering somewhat from the exclusive pursuits of production and consumption and toward a heightened concern with the quality of life (and hence, of health), then the demand for auxiliary workers to supplement the health professional will itself be unending. What the entry of the subprofessional or nonprofessional requires is a profound rethinking of health skills, roles, and statuses. A critical shortage of doctors, nurses, social workers, and administrators is very likely to be a permanent aspect of the health landscape. The established professions, then, must find avenues to extend their competence through collaboration with the less highly skilled, through far more precise definition of who can perform what job, and through inventive reorganization of the patterns of prevention and treatment.

Innovations in health care are shaping the roles of established and highly trained professionals toward a model of the consultant or supervisor or teacher rather than toward the active frontline practitioner. With such notable exceptions as surgery and public health nursing, the physician and nurse are cast increasingly often into administrative functions, into positions of seeing that care is given instead of giving it themselves. It should be remarked that the professional is all too commonly ill-prepared for this shift in roles, his technical skills being clinical rather than managerial. Thus we find an effort, especially in schools of public health and nursing, to build administrative and consultative talents into professional education. Further, the current emphasis on community health and the heavy participation of government at many levels in the health task mean that political knowledge and sensitivity are indispensable to the high-level professional.

Examples of the diversion of face-to-face care from the thoroughly accredited professional to varieties of auxiliary personnel are numerous. In mental health the need for staffing new community facilities is leading to the creation of a role for a "mental health assistant." This assistant is typically trained at a minimal level in the social sciences, with special emphasis on the conduct of interpersonal relations. He is not construed to be a qualified psychotherapist but a more modest helper and supporter for the psychologically distressed and, importantly, a source of referral to more expert, specialized helping agents. In general medical practice, again, experiment has begun with the role of "physician assistant." This individual will proceed from an intensive medical curriculum (but one far more brief than conventional medical training) to the functions of frontline care under an M.D.'s guidance.

An exceedingly important feature of the effort to establish auxiliary helping roles is that these positions are generally designed to be filled by persons who are roughly similar in social characteristics to their prospective clients. It is hoped that the auxiliaries will thereby do more than supply sheer manpower and will in fact help to close the gap between professional treater and lay client and to afford optimal use of leadership and skill in hitherto untapped sectors of the population.

CHAPTER 4

Medical Institutions

Like all organizations providing goods or services in American society, medical facilities exhibit the twin features of increasing complexity and increasing rationality. Their complexity stems from the great accretions of medical knowledge and technique that engender an ever-finer division of labor; too, medical institutions are subject to so many demands and expectations that they are, by definition, multiple in character. Their rationality, in turn, is a product of the imperatives of complex organizations for planning and control as well as the heightened imperative of economic accountability. Both complexity and rationality, however, despite being pervasive in modern organizational life, strike many critics as somehow alien in spirit to the helping relationship that is the crux of medical care. Thus the loose federation of many labors in a clinic is seen to threaten staff cohesion and patient wholeness; a complex patterning of services seems jarringly incongruous with the apparent simplicity of a human cry for help. And thus the rational exigencies of cost accounting or standardized personnel policies appear to deny the warmth and fervor of our empathic concern for one another.

But if medical institutions share with other enterprises these dominant structural themes, they are probably unique in the way they blend particular features of other, less comprehensive versions of institutional life. The hospital, for example, is at once a business, a hotel, a university, a social service agency, and so on through the long list of functions it is called on to perform. Hospitals resemble a business or factory in rapid flow of work, heavily practical emphasis on speedy results, and perhaps in the tangibility of desired outcome in levels of wellness. Yet they are very similar to the university in their array of specialists, their administrative confederation in a "collegial" bureaucracy (as distinguished from the "hierarchical" bureaucracy of business or governmental enterprise), and above all, in the fact that their product is people in a health process rather than a good or service once and finally delivered.

The General Hospital

If we select the hospital as the typical form of medical institution—and it is in many ways the central focus of contemporary health care—we can see represented in it most of the key characteristics of the human organization of medicine. These include comprehensiveness in time and space, the array of specialties, vulnerability to public scrutiny as an "open" setting, grouping of highly autonomous departments, parallel administrative and technical-medical lines of authority, physician dominance, and an ambivalent status in the eyes of those it serves, those who at once appreciate its healing hospitality and abhor the necessity of using it.

Hospitals, like doctors, have a long history of caretaking but only a relatively brief history of effective treatment of the ill. Until the early twentieth century the hospital was primarily a charitable organization that provided a setting in which the old, the homeless, the poor, and the friendless might die in minimal dignity. Going to the hospital represented a giving up, the terminal phase when nothing more could really be done for the afflicted; custodial support and tender loving care were the best that could be offered. Thus the mortality rates among patients *and* staff were truly staggering,[1] and anyone who could be cared

---

[1] "In 1788 the death rate among patients at the Hotel Dieu in Paris was 25 per cent, and that of surgeons and attendants from 6 to 12 per cent per annum." Temple Burling, Edith M. Lentz, and Robert

for in the household, especially the economically advantaged, shunned the hospital as a literal last resort. As late as the 1920s, hospital fund-raising appeals were often geared to a picture of the institution as an essentially charitable organization, a refuge for those who enjoyed no other. Only with the accelerated competence of modern medicine in our own era, when antiseptic, diagnostic, and surgical knowledge broke through the thick line of medical ignorance, did the hospital come to be seen as much in terms of hope as of horror. Only in the relatively recent past has the medical institution, rather than the home or the doctor's office, been construed as the physician's preferred workshop and the seat of miraculous cure.

The total caretaking that marked the hospital's historical role (and it is, of course, no accident that "hospital" and "hospitality" are commonly rooted) has now been joined by the elegance of therapeutic technique that makes this institution not just a comforter of life but a saver and giver of life. Hospitals are comprehensive in time; all hospital days contain twenty-four hours, and all hospital weeks contain seven days. Hospitals are likewise comprehensive in space, in at least two senses: they contain all necessary facilities under one roof, blanketing the patient's physical space, and they provide a total boundary for the inhabitant, blanketing his social space in an overarching environment. The hospital as "total institution," in Erving Goffman's telling phrase, remains the medical prototype, although there is currently a bubbling of experiment directed toward rendering it less total, toward opening it to the community and seeing it as just one link in a chain of helping services. Many mental hospitals, for instance, have installed the "unit system" in which patients from the same city or county are grouped together. This pattern not only serves to help maintain a sense of the individual's prehospital identity but also constitutes a focus for visiting and other activities by persons from the home community. The general hospital's permeability and linkage to the world outside its walls is emphasized in the development of home-treatment extension services and greatly expanded out-patient clinic facilities.

Medicine's exquisite division of labor, already remarked on

N. Wilson. *The Give and Take in Hospitals* (New York: Putnam, 1956), p. 4.

in the discussion of the health professions, flowers in the general hospital. The complexity of care implies a finely graded series of responsibilities and discrete tasks. Specialization means different things to the various parties in the medical transaction. To the patient it may mean that his care is fragmented, and he therefore feels there is no one he can talk to or who has responsibility for him as a total person. To the health professional specialization typically means that he has a niche of his own, a recognized role in treatment, and distressingly often, a competitive challenge in dealing with cospecialists. To the medical administrator this atomization of roles may present the gravest problems of coordination and continuity: How may the wealth of treaters be brought together for patient welfare and institutional stability? But there is clearly no turning back. The evolution of human enterprises seems always and everywhere to be in the direction of greater complexity, and so the issue is not to reverse specialization but to discover ways of accommodating it in coherent and well-focused patterns of health care.

Medical specialties, with their attendant scarce competencies and bristling prestige, tilt the forms of organization toward a grouping of independent units rather than toward a tight, unitary hierarchy. Hospitals tend to be federal systems without rigid central authority. Each department of the medical institution culivates its domains of activity, in treatment, research, teaching, or whatever, as a relatively autonomous fief. So the large general hospital, despite bearing one name and one spatial location, actually consists of the duchy of surgery, the principality of obstetrics, the free state of psychiatry, and so on. This system works reasonably (some might say astonishingly) well most of the time. Its twin defects are that interdepartmental collaboration in the patient's interest is problematic and that the hospital administrator finds it difficult to execute general organizational policy. The situation is remarkably parallel to that of operating an American university if students whose presenting symptom is ignorance be substituted for patients. On the other hand, disciplinary and departmental autonomy in medical settings generates a desirable "we-feeling," a sense of spirited freedom in the pursuit of expertness that is, on the whole, beneficial to both staff morale and patient care.

Problems of Authority

Closely woven into the pattern of professional autonomy, and the exaltation of technical skill, is the M.D.'s authoritative position in health affairs. Given the doctor's scientific and curative prestige and his legal responsibility for the patient's fate, it is perhaps understandable that he should also come to assume command over the organizational aspects of medical care. Yet his administrative dominance, only recently beginning to be questioned, is clearly unrelated to his therapeutic knowledge. Indeed, one might argue persuasively that the physician's very absorption in clinical detail, his concentration on the individual as a closed system of biological events, tends to make him unfit for that interpersonal and structural purview that is the essence of the administrative role. Nevertheless, the doctor has traditionally served as executive in medical institutions or at least as the power behind the layman or nurse who bore the formal executive title. Now, however, the complexity of organizations has given rise to the administrator-as-professional, to a specialization of the executive functions matching the specialization of healing functions. The thoroughly trained hospital or clinic administrator, if not yet quite an equal of the doctors on his staff, is approaching general equality and exerting mastery over the institution's modes of work.

The basic problem of split authority remains. No lay administrator can effectively dictate the course of bedside action or intrude into general clinical management. And neither can the physician, increasingly often, seriously pretend to master hospital personnel policy or the coordination of diverse independent departments. Administrative and medical lines of authority coexist in varying degrees of harmony or unease. If the conduct of war is too important to be left to the generals, the organization of medical care may be too important to be left to the physicians. But they must have a prominent voice. They must probably engage in a long-term dialectic with both medical administrators and concerned laymen.

Medical institutions have always been subject to public attitudes and pressures to a far greater extent than the business enterprise or most other institutional forms. The public, after all, enters directly into the organization as members of its clientele or as relatives and friends of the clientele. Further, the area of health seems naturally to be a more sensitive interest than are areas of commerce, education, and the like. Except for the desperately ill, who are for the moment aware only of the body and the chance of survival, sick people are probably more critical of the organizations that serve them, more irritable in the face of delay or disruption, than any other type of client. The eye of the social reformer falls eagerly on health services, for they are, almost by definition, inadequate in most places and times. Also, because better health care is an unquestioned good, he who agitates for medical reform can rely on broad support from salient human values. To all these forces must be added a growing public sophistication about medicine, spurred by higher levels of education and the widespread popularization of scientific novelty. The demand for health care, quantitative and qualitative, intensifies with the general societal raising of aspirations. The "revolution of rising expectations," which is characteristic of economic life in the developing countries, finds a counterpart in the great anticipations of the American people for medical efficacy.

That the public should adopt an ambivalent posture toward the hospital or clinic is not at all strange. People are grateful for help, but they naturally deplore the necessity of seeking it. Today, in addition to heightened expectations of medicine and the steady conquest of good health care as a fundamental human right, a more alert clientele fosters a closer analysis of the pathways entailed in the delivery of care. The political and economic constraints of federal legislation and third-party payers unquestionably imply an increased critical scrutiny of health practices. As George James, Dean of the Mt. Sinai School of Medicine, has observed, we are probably moving from a tradition of "producer-dominated" medicine into an era of "consumer-dominated" medicine. The concerned layman is becoming more heavily involved in health planning. This is in keeping with the realization that in the long run health can only be the entire community's business. Thus it is quite reasonable to anticipate not only that medical institutions will undergo vast changes in the near future but also that these changes will echo with the voices of the nonmedical public at least as loudly as with those of health professionals.

The Mental Hospital

Our examination of medical institutions has been confined to the model of the general hospital, especially the large multipurpose hospital. But this is obviously only one among many organizations designed to bring health resources and needful populations together. Indeed, the most dramatic attention of recent decades has been focused not on the general hospital but on the mental hospital. There are several excellent reasons for this concentration, among them the ghastly condition of the state hospitals, the well-publicized fact that mentally ill individuals occupy over half of all this nation's hospital beds, the immense costs of care, and perhaps, the inherent fascination that bizarre behavior exercises on the public imagination. (Note that "bizarre" behavior in mental hospitals has probably been as characteristic of organizational forms and organized treaters as it has of patients.) In addition, the winds of change have blown more strongly through our "human warehouses" in recent years than through any other medical institutions.

The general attributes of the public mental hospital are all too well known: geographic isolation from the community of the well; overcrowding and underbudgeting, with attendant outrages upon sanitation, diet, and privacy; the substitution of custodial care for any serious effort to treat illness; an emphasis on prisonlike conformity in an atmosphere of incarceration, accompanied at some times and places by punitive mistreatment; and abrogation of basic civil and human rights of the patient. Perhaps more damaging than the blatant horrors of the "snakepit" has been the insidious erosion of independence and self-regard brought about by enforced passivity and isolation. Thus were developed those "institutionalized personalities" who had learned the tasks of patienthood so thoroughly that they were forever unable to resume the normal social roles of the mentally well. Consigned by society to a limbo, the long-term patient learned to live in what amounted to a social vacuum. He came to adapt his aspirations and behaviors to the patterns most agreeable to the staff and achieved a sort of expertness in the condition of being hospitalized.

There were, of course, a set of very familiar reasons why all this should be so. Public sentiments about psychological disorders had historically stressed the dangers threatened by the floridly ill, and hence the community's urgent desire to locate mental patients out of sight and out of mind. Not only did people fear the mentally disturbed individual, but his condition was typically attended by an air of hopelessness. In the absence of any clear-cut biological agent of disease (or at any rate, the failure to identify any such etiological villain) for most varieties of disorder, the public felt rightly that comparatively little could be done for the patient. Understaffing meant that a given patient's contact with any physician was minimal. Treatment was for the most part custodial rather than curative, the latter consisting of sporadic organic efforts such as shock therapy or occasional psychotherapeutic encounters.

Since World War II, however, and especially in the last decade, two strands of truly revolutionary change in the mental hospital have appeared. The first of these was actually a revival of certain ideas and values that had surfaced at least once before, in the "moral treatment" of nineteenth-century reform. This was essentially a recognition of the disturbed person as a human being who possesses a valid claim to dignity and a genuine potential for return to normalcy. Premised on the assumption that individuals who are treated as fully human and are engaged in sequences of normal interpersonal relations by those around them will indeed behave normally for the most part, this shift in orientation was accompanied by increased attention to the social structure of the mental institution. A series of fresh psychological and sociological investigations revealed the existence of a patient culture as well as a staff culture and showed how the hospital constituted a total system of relationships that had meaning for each patient's chance of improvement. Erving Goffman brilliantly traced the patient's "career" in the hospital, and his work implied that that dismal career might be altered or interrupted. Alfred Stanton and Morris Schwartz and William Caudill pointed out that all the events in the hospital system were influential on patients' states of health. Otto Von Mering and Stanley King and Esther Lucille Brown explored the tendency for hospitals to change from primarily custodial to importantly therapeutic organizations. In all, there arose a renewed conviction that attentive care, utilizing the full resources of staff culture and patient culture, might reclaim a major fraction of those who had been cast aside by their society. Intensive therapeutic efforts even demonstrated some signal, if partial, victories among the populations of the notorious "back wards," the habitat of the most deteriorated long-stay patients.

The second revolutionary strand, complementing the first with an appropriateness seldom found in human affairs, was the emergence of chemotherapeutic technique. Tranquilizers and energizers provide for the first time a lever for the control of symptoms, and to some extent, of mood, that enables treatment to go forward in something approaching calm rationality. Whether or not the "core" of the illness, the underlying conflicts and predispositions that are postulated by psychodynamic theory, is ever effectively altered, the individual is at least enabled to perform standard social roles with some efficiency. This attainment of minimal functional competence accounts for a changed, more hopeful atmosphere in the hospital, much more speedy discharge, and the possibility of maintaining large numbers of ill people at home in their community. It fits nicely into the emphasis on active therapy and on the interactive engagement of the patient; in brief, the disturbed individual can be chemotherapeutically "fitted" for interpersonal relatedness.

The Hospital in the Community

Along with the thrust toward actively helping and the physical stabilization through drugs that enables the patient to take part in his treatment, a movement toward lowering the wall between the mental hospital and its environing society has also been present. The wall is still up, but it has been breached in several places: patients are encouraged to visit the community; the public, as well as relatives, has been emphatically invited in; and community facilities, such as out-patient clinics and general hospitals, are more often tied to the mental hospital in a coherent network of services. There is, too, an effort to overcome the great size and "mass" character of the state hospital, both by building smaller institutions and by splitting up large ones into manageable units.

All the attempts to blur institutional lines and provide helping services for the mentally ill in a manner more appropriate to patient need than to bureaucratic tradition are a part of the current sustained push toward a true community medicine. Linking facilities together and centering them on the patient's natural social milieu is becoming more characteristic of health services in general, not only in the mental health field. For example, the partial hospitalization of the "day hospital" (or "night hospital") in which a patient may leave the institution to carry on usual work or familial roles has its general medical counterpart in such arrangements as home visiting care or "meals on wheels."

The steady repatterning of medical institutions to make them more firmly a part of total community life and more directly accessible to the place and time of population health needs is illustrated by many contemporary innovations. These will be examined in more detail in Chapter 5. They include the greatly expanded mandate of public health departments, the articulation of public with private resources, the establishment of comprehensive community mental health centers, and the burgeoning of health planning as a recognized local responsibility. In effect, the massive federal support of health care is forcing medical institutions to lodge themselves solidly in their local social systems and to be more responsive to total population demands for care. In turn, public consciousness of health matters and public assumption of a heavy influence on institutional arrangements are tending toward a conception of health as "everybody's" business and not as solely the business of medical professionals or medical institutions. We can quite confidently expect a ferment of organizational change in the next few years as our society at last turns upon the delivery of health care with the same rational attention and experimental inclination that has marked our approaches to clinical medical research. That genius for problem solving that hitherto has been largely restricted to industrial production and to investigation in the physical and natural sciences is at length beginning to focus on what were once the frills of our national life. The needs of people for helping services in health and education are moving from marginal to central concerns of American life in the late twentieth century. Medicine will be really *in* society as never before and *in* in the most urgent and exciting fashion.

CHAPTER 5

The Community
Framework

Health may be viewed, as we have done in the last several chapters, in the context of doctor-patient relations, professional activities, and the organization of roles into medical institutions. However, the processes of health and illness and society's efforts to cope with them are probably best seen in the more comprehensive framework of the population living group: the community. There are many convincing reasons for choosing the community as a focus of analysis. Chief among them are two, one concerning the causal network that generates illness and one dealing with the goals of preventing and curing illness.

In the realm of cause we are growing more and more aware that most of the health states presenting serious risks are multicausal in nature. Because these illnesses are not entirely explainable in terms of a single etiological agent attacking the organism, in the fashion suggested by the classical germ theory of disease, we now search for patterns of causal factors that fit together to produce pathology. This search entails exploration of a range of processes, from the level of the microorganism to the level of man's culturally phrased designs for living. Only in the thorough embeddedness of man-in-community, the human population moving through family, school, work, and neighborhood, can such multiple exploration be well carried out. Thus the disorganization of the ghetto has more to do with mild mental retardation than do any number of predisposing genetic factors. Impoverishment and lack of prenatal care, characteristic of crowded nonwhite areas in large cities (and many uncrowded rural areas), betray the links between community structure and the rates of infant mortality. The major categories of death and disability can only be comprehended in a community focus.

When we try to stave off or alleviate sickness, when we try to deliver medical resources to those groups most in need of them, it once again is apparent that the mustering of care is intimately attached to community structure. A recent publication bears the title, *Health Is a Community Affair* (Cambridge, Mass.: Harvard University Press, 1967). So it is, and the overriding problem of modern public health is to discover ways of mobilizing the community for a concerted attack, lay and professional, upon health deficits. Prevention and treatment involve the total local scene in two main guises. First, an appropriate organization of services demands a close knowledge of local health problems and of the variety of local helping agents. Second, the approach to target populations necessarily entails substantial knowledge of how these populations live—their styled group behavior—and how they regard health and helpers—their styled responses to medical professionals and to their own health conditions. Both living habits and health perceptions are clearly based in peoples' experience of living together in time and space. Therefore, the delivery of care depends upon recognition of the social systems involved, of the fitting together of groups in that patterned, durable relatedness termed "community."

Workers in public health cherish a trite but noble maxim that "the community is the patient." This phrase presumably means that instead of orienting health services to the individual considered alone, a medical professional should direct his first attention to the health of populations considered in their total social settings. It may also be taken to imply an exceedingly broad medical mandate, as in Edward McGavran's assertion that public health "is nothing more or less than a scientific approach to the diagnosis and treatment of the body politic—the history, the physical examination, the tests, the analysis, the clinical judgment, and the prescription for treatment." [1] The very sweeping nature of the mandate raises certain difficult questions. So, too, does the perilous analogy between the individual-as-organism and the community-as-organism. Although it is quite true that society, like the body, is composed of interdependent systems and that events occurring in any given system reverberate in other subsystems, we must recognize that mutuality among sectors of a community is far less thoroughgoing than the pervasive mutuality of body processes. Further, we must beware of imagining that communities possess anything approaching the central nervous system, either in singleness of purpose or unitary mechanisms of control.

Yet the image of community-as-patient is dramatically stimulating and may well afford a springboard for closer analysis of the health context. We might profitably direct several inquiries to the implications of this provocative analogy. Three such central questions, shockingly obvious but often unexamined, are:

1. If the community is the patient, *what kind* of patient is it?
2. If the community is the patient, *whose* patient is it?
3. If the community is the patient, *how* may it be treated most effectively?

What Kind of Patient is the Community?

Attempts to define the community are legion; the history of speculation about how men can live in concert dates at least from Plato's observations about an ideal social order and Aristotle's theories of politics. Contemporary interest in a definition is as timely as the latest census findings or the effort to mobilize the "community of the poor" in the war on poverty. Broadly speaking, concepts about the community's essential nature may be grouped as geographic ecological or social psychological.

Geographic ecological approaches stress such defining criteria as population density, economic interdependence, centralization of transport and shopping facilities, and natural geographic clustering around topographic features. They tend to label as a

[1] Edward G. McGavran, "The Scientific Diagnosis and Treatment of the Community of the Patient," *Public Health News*, 38 (February 1958), 61–68.

community that aggregation of people who interact with one another more often than with residents of "outside" areas and who depend upon one another for those goods and services that sustain everyday life.

Social psychological approaches likewise emphasize interaction rates—the frequency of contact—in their model of the community. They are further concerned with the institutionalized interdependence of people enacting social roles, with what might be termed a complementarity of activity. This matching of peoples' expectations of one another, the root symmetry on which social systems rest, is not confined to the economic or political spheres but extends into health, recreation, and varieties of other human enterprises. Perhaps most distinctive in a social psychological vein is the assumption that members of a community embrace certain common values and share a feeling of belonging or identity with a specific population grouping.

The most conventional means of determining a community (and an exceedingly useful one for many purposes) is to seek out established political divisions. Although such lines of governmental authority are often not consonant with either of the major perspectives sketched above, these formal channels must be understood and worked with to accomplish most practical outcomes in health or any other sphere. In part, our enforced reliance on political definitions inheres in the fact that the political system is the locus of legitimate authority, empowered to sanction the directions of local action. In part, too, the political manifold is integral to the allocation of group resources, to the expenditure of public monies for ends on which some measure of local consensus has been reached. Yet the ordinary domains of government jurisdiction may be radically unsuited to either the diagnosis or the treatment of community health; political classifications may be *mis*classifications of population health needs or habits. For example, an increasingly frequent theme in regional health planning is the analysis of "health trade areas," regions that seemingly form natural clusters of health problems and service facilities. These health trade areas are commonly found to leap over the traditional political boundaries, often embracing several corporate units, counties, or even sections of two states. Clearly, then, under these legal conditions, it is hard to achieve concerted planning or consistent strategy. In a more general sense, the multiplicity and overlapping of political jurisdictions —from the township to the federal government—generates confusion in any rational attempt to confront health problems. Coordination of governmental levels and sectors becomes a major issue in coping with health's community framework. In this respect, of course, medicine is not at all unique because the fragmentation of political authority bedevils all who would mount programs of social action in the contemporary United States.

These alternative ways of defining a community reflect reality: the concept is complex. But because definition guides action, the worker in community medicine must essay some minimal outline for health purposes. He must at least try to determine *what kind* of patient he is dealing with when he approaches the community. Any outline is perforce incomplete. One can never know "enough" about any human population to be perfectly assured that he understands its patterns of behavior or that he can effectively collaborate with a local human organization to enact desired change.

Probably the first considerations to be emphasized are that the community is a *system of relationships* and that each community is in important respects *unique*. We must conceive of the community as a system in order to assess the influence of one part upon another and to see that both health needs and our responses to them are multidetermined by interlocking features of the whole. One must apprehend the particularities of local situations if he is to avoid the egregious error of assuming that some mechanical model of community structure will allow him to transfer knowledge and techniques blindly from one setting to another.

Recognizing communities as systems of relationships immediately directs our attention to the various parts of the structure and to how they influence one another. This conception drives us to ask, What are the most significant political, economic, medical, and other institutions? Who are the most influential persons manning the institutional patterns? How is the population subdivided by age, sex, race, ethnicity, and socioeconomic status? What are the paramount health needs? and How are these needs distributed in this population? Recognizing local uniqueness fastens our interest on the specific lineaments of community history and most especially on the story of how the population has be-

haved in past encounters with health or other critical problems.
Above all, the stress on what is characteristic of *this* locale's "personality" enhances our appreciation of the designs for living—the
culture—that have to be known before we can sensibly link
cause and effect in the production of disease or the habitual response to disease.

Thus a profile of its major characteristics is essential to an
informed view of the community-as-patient. A sophisticated social survey, in as much depth as possible, is a prerequisite to
community medicine. Only in this fashion, somewhat analogous
to the medical history of the individual patient, can events be
placed in context. And only when we possess a reasonable community baseline can we attempt to measure the consequences of
public health action.

Finally, despite our stress on the unique properties of a given
community, it is vital to realize that no contemporary community
in the United States is a self-contained entity. The student of
community health must consistently be aware of the multiple ties
between any local area and the larger surrounding society and of
the fact that neither its problems nor its resources lend themselves to a parochial analysis. Water or air pollution, heart disease, or mental illness are not generated or enclosed within local
boundaries. Also, the talents and budgets necessary to attack
them are seldom discovered within a single home district. We
live in a society that is exquisitely interdependent and one, moreover, that is seeing regional differences increasingly blurred by
adherence to a prevailing middle class culture.

Whose Patient is the Community?

In the last analysis it is probably true that the community is
"its own" patient, that only a mustering of total local resources,
voluntary and governmental, can cope with complex health problems. Yet to term the total community both patient *and* doctor is
probably excessively metaphorical, not to say outrageously opti-
mistic. Even if nearly all members of the population might be
persuaded to become conscious of health and willing to help,
some much smaller, specialized number would remain primarily
responsible for health action.

These local health leaders and practitioners, in whose charge the community now rests uneasily but must, for better or worse, rest, may be divided into three major varieties. They might be termed *the public or governmental system of care, the private system of care,* and *the lay system of concern.* Much of the energy spent in current health planning and indeed in most everyday medical activity is necessarily devoted to yoking these three forces into some reasonable working arrangement. Our society, and developed industrial societies in general, have been overtaken by the intensity of interdependence. Although a pronounced mutuality among the different sectors of the population, both in generating health needs and devising responses to those needs, has always been present, the mutuality is greatly heightened today by the industrial division of labor, ease of transport and communication, swelling population, and the increasingly urban character of the society. Especially in a nation like our own, long wedded to values of individualism and laissez-faire in health matters (as in much else), the awareness of interdependence is slow in taking hold. It is one thing to embrace the maxim that one is his brother's keeper as an ideal and freely chosen virtue; it is quite another to be faced with the same proposition as an imperative, as an iron law of survival. The novelist Peter De Vries puts the situation bluntly in his aphorism that we are not placed in this world for seeing through one another but for seeing one another through.

Given the fact of interdependence, what do the three great helping systems whose patient is the community actually perform? A brief answer must surely be that they perform a very great deal but that the health yield is disjunctive, ill-coordinated, and insufficient. The public governmental system offers a plethora of services to the disadvantaged strata and increasingly to many other population groups as well. These range from the medical care given in a Veterans Administration hospital to research on air pollution or mental illness to the everyday operations of the local health department in environmental sanitation or family-based nursing. The private sector not only delivers superior care to that part of the population who can pay for services but also, of course, contributes to the common weal through a series of free (or low-cost) facilities and through health research. The lay system of concern, which in most communities is actually a mixed lay and professional grouping, is intricately involved in activities running from hospital trusteeship to participation in voluntary associations, such as a mental health association, to concerted planning and study for the knitting together of local facilities. More and more frequently, as we have noted, this lay system is pressing, and being pressed, to assume the huge task of health planning. The task, to be sure, is not done in isolation from the public or private health professional cadres and institutions. Yet it *is* devolving on substantial numbers of local leaders who typically have scant medical knowledge and often scant knowledge of community processes but who are achieving a rapid and forced sophistication in such matters.

Our answer to the question, Whose patient is the community? thus rests on the array of public, voluntary, and lay resources. At least two substantial issues arise when the public health is viewed in this total network of helping agents. The first concerns the respective domains assigned to or preempted by the various care facilities. Is the health of the total community solely the charge of public agencies? If not, as the consensus of informed opinion now increasingly often asserts, how can medical facilities be linked together in an intelligible style? If community health levels are "everybody's" business, then the division of labor required to improve them can only be brought about by free negotiation or by directive fiat or by some combination of these modes.

The alternative of free negotiation may be seen in the operation of what sociologists Sol Levine and Paul White have termed "exchange" processes. Here, the various agencies involved in local health action develop willy-nilly a form of reciprocity in which they essentially trade off clients and functions. They agree, formally or informally, to respect one another's chosen special domains and to make referrals of clients conform to those domains. In the pattern of medicine in this country, there are few precedents for or examples of integration of services by fiat. What is now emerging, however, is a mixed model (consonant with the pattern of most important enterprises in the society as a whole) that entails a combination of government directive—especially in setting criteria of care and of payment for care—with both voluntary exchange and lay health planning. Whether the result of the combination is an integrated system of care or a haphazard jumble of overlapping facilities varies from community to community. It is probably fair to say that the jury is still out, that in the present phase of experiment, achievement, and error, we really do not know how to construct a workable mosaic of services.

The second intrusive issue, not unrelated to that of coordination and integration, pivots on the distribution of professional versus lay authority. We have noted several contradictory threads affecting this distribution of authority: the physician's spot at the apex of medical power; the demands of other medical professionals and health administrators to share this power; the growing disposition of lay leadership—political, economic, and intellectual—to exert a potent influence in health affairs. In the potential conflict between expert and amateur versions of the desirable, American medicine is rehearsing a much more general theme that affects modern societies, the calculus Sir Alfred Zimmern phrased as "the right relation between knowledge and power." We have historically hemmed in the expert's discretion in matters of fundamental policy, as distinguished from those decisions that seem more purely technical. Thus nominally, and to a considerable extent actually, experts in the top echelons of government are subject to veto and final choice by administrative generalists, that is, by political figures in executive and legislative branches. Yet because the grounds for decision making today are so often pervaded by highly technical considerations, there is a genuine question about the efficacy, and indeed the possibility, of continuing lay dominance. There are many familiar illustrations, dating especially from the rise of physicists and engineers to heavily influential advisory roles in World War II.

In a sense, medicine shows a reverse process: it has arrived at lay-expert balancing by the opposite path. Questions about health have almost always been assumed to lie in the health professional's province. Only in our own time, when community and national health decisions have truly entered the arena of public policy, has the expert become importantly subject to the kind of embarrassing inquiry that presidents direct to admirals or that company executives direct to chief chemists. No community leader is apt to challenge a surgeon about the proper procedures for open-heart surgery. Physicians and other health workers may well be challenged, however, about patterns for the organization of medical facilities or priorities in the allocation of research monies. And it is in such contexts that the struggle between schooled professional and newly alerted layman may be joined.

How May the Community be Treated?

How may the community-as-patient be treated most effectively? Part of the answer, surely, lies in the way we answer the two earlier questions (*What kind* of patient is it? and *Whose* patient is it?). Our discussion thus far suggests that the community must be treated as a whole, as an interdependent system of social relationships, because it is that kind of patient. Further, it should be treated comprehensively, by an integrated network of services, because the community is the patient of several classes of agents. Most significantly, the question of how to treat a community provokes an interest in the timing and the setting of care.

Public health professionals are at one in insisting on the importance of timing. Health costs and general social costs are minimized when the community is treated early. Ideally, as the stress on "primary" prevention indicates, treatment begins before any disease processes are visible. Population wellness is best sustained when healthful living patterns can be fostered from the very beginning of the life cycle, in fact, from before the beginning of any individual's life, in the behavior of his parents. Health and illness, like life itself, are cumulative.

Viewing health problems in a community framework, we can clearly see that the levels of functioning sought for large population groups are far more dependent upon the total style of behavior in which those groups are caught up than on a clinical grappling with individual cases of disorder. The telling examples of this proposition are all around us, notably in the massive evidence of a broad relationship between poverty and various states of ill health. An enabling, a lifting, of the economically and culturally deprived sectors of the community would unquestionably do more for a range of pathology, from mental illness to venereal disease, than any number of clinics or drugs. Unfortunately, prevention and treatment at later stages of the pathological chain, when frank illness is incarnate in particular individuals, are both more comfortably appropriate to social conventions and more surely achievable in a technical sense. Primary prevention—fostering health and anticipating disease—really asks of society a kind of commitment to community management and deliberative change that is historically alien to American culture. Yet there are fairly loud signals saying that our reluctance to attempt prevention at the root of disease processes, rather than dealing solely with dead or crippled branches, is being overcome. From the well-baby clinic to school mental health to the war on poverty itself, there are tangible indications that our sense of community timing is growing more accurate.

If genuinely primary prevention is seldom achieved, community medicine has nevertheless exerted pressure on the timing of health events so that *early* intervention in illness ("secondary" prevention) is much more frequent. Two familiar illustrations of early intervention are tuberculosis screening by means of chest X-rays and other techniques and timely detection of cancer of the uterus through cervical smears. In each of these instances, as in many others that might be cited, intervention is based on a community-wide orientation. The appeal for detection is addressed to population groups and is increasingly shrewdly tailored to specific patterns of belief and behavior in those groups. We shall analyze modes of population response to preventive and early treatment efforts in Chapter 8.

The third chronological phase, so-called tertiary prevention, is directed toward enabling people to recover from episodes of illness or to live reasonably while continuing to manifest a chronic disease. Here again, community-based avenues of care are increasingly the treatments of choice. Thus we find a thrust toward caring for the aged and the chronically ill in their own households or in intermediate facilities, such as nursing homes, that stand partway between "complete" medical institutions and normal households. Many general hospitals, as well as public health departments, are engaged in the struggle to maintain patients at home. In the field of mental health, especially, we now observe a concerted push to fix all three varieties of timing in an appropriate community setting: primary prevention in home and school, encouraging competent interpersonal behavior; secondary prevention at many points, from the "walk-in" clinic to the general hospital, trying to stave off the exacerbation of symptoms into frank breakdown; tertiary prevention in the home, the day hospital, or the sheltered workshop, attempting to bring the ex-mental hospital patient back into the local fabric of social organization.

Our discussion of timing has largely implied its corollary emphasis in the community framework, namely the social setting of health care. One might say there are two kinds of "closeness" involved in the quest for local efficacy: health professionals wish to intervene at a point in time as close as possible to the presumed beginning of the causal chain(s) of illness, and they also wish the scene of health action to be as close as possible in physical and social space to the normal living environment of the population. Simply, one answer to how to treat a community is: treat it where it is, where people live, so that health care forms a natural element of ongoing life processes.

There are several sound reasons for stressing that the health setting be integral to the community. On strictly medical criteria, it has generally been found that care is more effective and briefer when the patient is confronted in his customary milieu rather than ripped away from this scene and placed in the artificially closed environment of the hospital. Except for certain acute situations, the transition from home to hospital and back again may add an important social psychological disruption to the disruption of the illness as such. In addition, in some of the chronic and especially mental diseases, prolonged hospitalization may ill-equip a patient for a return to his usual social roles; he is at risk of developing an institutionalized personality that is at sharp variance with the demands of the world outside the hospital. There are also thought to be treatment benefits in the supportive atmosphere of kin and familiar associates, although, of course, such increments depend upon the tone of relatedness already established in the household and other settings. Finally, health action that occurs literally within the community may make for a more economical use of professional manpower and may inspire a wider vigilance in health matters on the part of the general pub-'ic.

From the Inside:
Sociology in Medicine

Part One dealt with medicine and society as they might be seen by a curious outside observer. It placed the social scientist in the position of a relatively detached analyst, interested in what goes on in the world of health but not directly implicated as a participant in health enterprises.

The role of sociology in Part Two is rather different. Here we are not content to gaze coolly at the behavior of doctors and patients or at the organization of medical facilities. Instead, we wish to inquire, as fellow professionals in health, into the relationships between certain social and psychological factors and a series of medical problems. These problems are of two main varieties: the production of states of illness and the mounting of strategies for coping with them. The two concerns correspond to the major emphases of modern social medicine or social epidemiology. We are interested in discovering where illness occurs in human populations as a prelude to investigating why it should occur in this group and not in that one. Then, in complementary fashion, we want to explore society's reactions to the facts of ill health. In particular, we seek knowledge of why people do or do not lend themselves to programs of prevention or treatment designed by medical professionals. In each of these areas, our main interest will be to assess the ways in which man's social behavior —his relations to other people and to himself in vital life sectors, such as familial and occupational roles—influences his chances of staying well, becoming ill, or responding to health care. Throughout, we shall attempt to join peoples' ways of life to their ways of health.

CHAPTER 6

The Distribution
of Illness[1]

If states of ill health were randomly distributed in human populations, we should have to assume either that illness is simply inherent in being human (a proposition that contains a fair measure of truth) or that illness is invariably caused by a uniformly patterned attack by "outside" agents, such as germs, that are no respecters of individual differences. But, of course, health is not so distributed. Health and illness appear very unevenly arrayed across a variety of classifications of populations. It is precisely the differential occurrence of health conditions that piques scientific curiosity and supplies the elementary clues in the search for cause.

Comparison of Populations

In nineteenth-century clinical medicine one of the great scientific leaps was the simulation of experimental methods by the

---

[1] Many of the basic data for this chapter are drawn from the extremely useful summary by Monroe Lerner and Odin W. Anderson, *Health Progress in the United States* (Chicago: The University of Chicago Press, 1965).

method of case comparisons. Indeed, some investigators rigged a quasi-experimental model by placing in adjoining hospital beds two individuals who were similar in most respects but different in the criteria of interest. It then remained to observe how a distinction in some feature of treatment or in some characteristic of the patient was connected to a specifiable distinction in health outcome. Contemporary epidemiology consists in large part of extending the comparative model to sizeable groups of people, to populations that are alike in major features but dissimilar in some crucial respects, in having substantially different rates of an illness, for example. Then the investigator proceeds to ask a series of questions, to the end of ferreting out what differing characteristics in the two groups accompany the observed differences in their health. The characteristics that distinguish the two groups range very widely, from seemingly clear-cut differences like age or sex or place of residence to apparently much more subtle variations of psychological state or social circumstance. The differences, on occasion, may reside in what look like trivial alterations of daily behavior, of the habits of living.

The importance of contrasting distributions of illness in spurring the approach to cause and hence to control is vividly exemplified in one of the classic epidemiological studies, the work of John Snow on cholera in Victorian London. Snow, an especially observant and meticulous physician, kept track of the geographic location of cholera cases in the metropolis. Not only did he plot when and where cases were reported, but he also carefully inquired into the routine behavior of the victims—where they had journeyed, what they had eaten and drunk, and so on. Even though he lacked a well-developed causal hypothesis (in fact, the cholera vibrio—the specific disease agent—had not yet been discovered), Snow began to suspect that the illness was conveyed by water, and he was shrewd enough to array his cases according to where they got their water supply as well as to where they lived. London of that day was served by several water companies, some that piped water from relatively pure sources and others that pumped water from contaminated sources. Snow, after plotting the occurrence of cholera cases, concluded that contaminated water might account for their distribution. In the now legendary and symbolic act that marked one of the first triumphs of epidemiology and public health,

Snow removed the handle of the Broad Street Pump and cholera attacks declined among its former users. (Although Snow's *method* of detection is a model of epidemiological research, the *history* of the cholera epidemic is somewhat more complicated than this brief sketch suggests. Actually, the rate of attack had begun to decline even before Snow closed the pump.)

Unfortunately, the most prominent health problems in today's developed, industrialized societies do not lend themselves to ready solution by such dramatic interventions as Snow's. They are by and large disorders of a quite different sort than cholera. Rather than infectious or communicable diseases in which some specific, primary microorganismic agent is present, the chief killers and disablers are what we might call "dis-eases of living." They include a variety of chronic and degenerative ills, complemented by derangements in man's relation to his human and manmade environment. Leading causes of death and disability in advanced industrial societies include heart disease, cancer, accidents, and mental illness. Even those health states that still bulk large in importance and in which a specific pathogenic agent *is* at hand—tuberculosis and venereal disease, for instance—are known to depend heavily on social and psychological events that encourage or deter the onset of illness.

In contrast, the developing and undeveloped nations show a sharply different pattern of major health hazards. In those societies the "traditional" diseases of human history, based in transmission of identified disease agents and exacerbated by poor sanitation and malnutrition, remain prominent. Thus the first notable distinction in how diseases are distributed among population groups becomes apparent when we place the health profiles of rich countries beside the profiles of poor countries or, perhaps more accurately, the health profiles of industrialized societies beside the profiles of unindustrialized societies. One does not, of course, find a perfect symmetry: malnutrition is present both in Mississippi and in New York City and cancer can be found in rural Africa. But the main pattern is clear, so clear that many observers believe we may see a regular sequence of health problems unfolding in step with a country's shift in social organization from rural to urban and from agricultural to industrial.

One type of evidence to support the idea that a society's position on a scale of urbanization-industrialization is closely related to its characteristic diseases is this comparison of advanced nations with less advanced ones. For example, health levels and types of current problems are remarkably convergent among a cluster of advanced countries. Infant mortality rates, life expectancy, and major causes of death are roughly similar for the United States, Sweden, England, and France. Uniformly, communicable disease is low as a source of death and chronic disease is high. These are all countries, although obviously not the only ones, where the accomplishments of scientific medicine and public health have taken hold with massive effect. Another type of evidence stems from the comparison of health profiles at different points in time within a single country. The United States is a convenient, well-documented example. In 1900 the leading causes of death were such illnesses as infant diarrhea, pneumonia, and tuberculosis. In 1960 the ranking had shifted so that coronary heart disease, cancer, cerebral-vascular diseases, and accidents led the list.

The pace of industrial development and the movement to city living are surely not the only accompaniments to such drastic changes in the distribution of health. Heavily implicated is the progress of the health sciences themselves. With the exception of accidents, and here the rise of the automobile is a significant contributor, most of the major causes of death and disability are in one sense the kinds of hazards that overtake the individual who has been kept alive long enough to encounter them. That is, they tend to be the degenerative ills of aging; they attack large numbers of people who presumably would have succumbed during an earlier period of history at younger ages. Having been preserved from infection, communicable disease, and the random insults of a less hygienic environment, the individual is felled at last by internal erosion. As Iago Galdston, a pioneering figure in social medicine, once put it, colorfully if a bit cryptically, the dance of death has lengthened but its measure remains the same. This proposition is further buttressed by the fact that, at a given time in the United States, there are significant health differences between wealthy industrial regions and poor agricultural ones. In overall mortality rates, for example, there is a substantial differential favoring "high income" states, such as the urban industrial Northeast, as opposed to "low income" states, such as most of the South. The margin is especially marked in infant mortality. Further, mortality from the chronic diseases—heart ailments and cancer—shows just the reverse pattern: the ills of modern living are unevenly concentrated in wealthy states.

These gross differences in the distribution of illness have vital implications both for the search for causal factors and for efforts to improve people's health. Beyond the general distinctions between industrial and nonindustrial societies, there are a large number of contrasts internal to a given society. Such contrasts point up the uneven clustering of health problems and life chances among members of varying groups. The most interesting and provocative differences in the contemporary United States ("gradients of risk," in the technical tongue of epidemiology) are those associated with the characteristics of *age, sex, race,* and *socioeconomic rank.*

Age

The striking increase in life expectancy and decline of mortality in the United States in the recent past reflect primarily a great triumph over the risks of childbearing and the diseases of infancy and childhood. Once past the earliest days of life, people are at greatly decreased risk of dying until they advance into the degenerative exposure of the middle years. The single major exception to this assurance of a healthy childhood and young adulthood is found in the high mortality rate from accidents among young adult men. Obviously, the risks of dying or becoming ill advance steadily with increasing age. Yet this heightened risk at older ages is not solely of interest as a matter of biological decay; the distribution of illness by age leads us as well into a series of social and psychological questions. What ordinary stresses in the wear and tear of living a life bear most heavily on the aging individual? What accumulations of pressures from family life, work life, or the pace of an urban environment pile up on the person? Is the effect of air and water pollution, noise, smoking, and drinking only demonstrably pathogenic after a cumulative exposure? Which specific hazards attached to the social role of the older person are most probably deleterious: loosening of interpersonal bonds with children, loss of friends, isolation, or retirement and attendant feelings of uselessness? Thus to know that the single characteristic, "age," seemingly the simplest of all categories for classifying population groups, is related to systematic differences in health rates implies a host of clues for etiological search. It also implies, of course, myriad questions of individual posture and social policy in the care of the aged.

Sex

Sex differences in illness and death are extremely significant in American society. The most striking single generalization is that women are very much advantaged in life expectancy. Male death rates exceed female death rates at all ages and for all causes except diabetes. For instance, in 1959 female babies enjoyed an average of six and one-half years more life expectancy than male babies. Although mortality rates for the population as a whole have declined importantly in the past fifty years, the decline has been less for men than for women. Deaths are concentrated by cause in those categories in which males are at heightened risk, such as heart disease and accidents.

Men suffer their substantial health inferiority from the combined impact of two major patterns of cause: the biological and the social psychological. That the male of the species is in fact the weaker sex is demonstrable from earliest life: males show excess mortality even in the prenatal and neonatal periods. The male is more vulnerable *as organism* even in the era before any exposure to differential stress in life situations can begin to take hold. Social psychological factors that influence male health adversely are presumed to be of several kinds. The argument for their operation is at this point merely plausible and not conclusive because research in social epidemiology is still an infant enterprise. An example of increased male exposure to socially shaped hazards is seen in accident rates. Because accidents are a major source of excess male deaths, it is appropriate to inquire into the sex differences in risk. A range of fairly obvious factors may be supposed, centering around contrasting sex roles in key areas of life, especially the occupational. Men in our society are expected, in general, to be aggressive in work and play. High accident rates among younger men may be attributed to their exposure to risks in sports, outdoor activity of all kinds, dangerous occupations, and so on. But one suspects that these risks are exaggerated by social role pressures that reward impulsiveness and resolute activism; younger males in automobiles are perhaps the most dramatic illustration. It might be important, also, to explore the psychodynamics of male competitiveness, both in all-male peer groups and in situations involving females. Socially, men are defined as aggressors, risk takers, and doers of dirty or life-threatening jobs. Psychologically, they may engage the world in terms that blur the distinction between physical courage and foolhardy exposure.

Another prominent body of evidence for social environmental factors in excess male mortality is seen in the fact that the sex differences in death rates are most pronounced in larger cities and higher occupational groups. This suggests that certain life styles may exert an unequally heavy stress on men. We cannot say what it is about tense urban living or executive or professional work responsibilities that bears down especially hard on men. Such differences in life chances, however, are provocative and spur the quest for social cause. The male, then, is more vulnerable *as social actor,* and this compounds his biological handicaps. Altogether, there is persuasive support for the familiar statement among health professionals that the group at greatest risk in the United States today is middle-aged males.

Sex differences in self-reported illness are just the reverse of the mortality picture. Women consistently exhibit higher morbidity than men. Illness rates are, of course, far less reliable data than are death rates, because the latter can be fairly confidently enumerated in an advanced industrial society, whereas the former are subject to all kinds of distortion in definition and reporting. Nevertheless, surveys of populations repeatedly show females reporting larger numbers of symptoms and more episodes of illness. The reason may be that the act of defining oneself as ill, and perhaps even of explicitly recognizing some types of symptoms, is more appropriate to the social role of the woman than to that of the male. Women would appear to have the best of both worlds, to enjoy advantages coming and going. They are biologically more fit, less often exposed to physical and social psychological hazards, and then take better care of themselves if they *should* fall ill. There is also the distinct possibility that at least certain sorts of mortality and morbidity may run in opposite patterns, so that being a little ill quite often is protective for women, whereas Spartan males go on to collapse finally and comprehensively in the fashion of Oliver Wendell Holmes' one-horse shay.

Uneven distributions of death and sickness between the sexes suggest many avenues of inquiry. Why does the male begin life with a biological handicap? What are the especially hazardous features of men's occupational and familial roles? What aspects of the woman's life space induce her higher reported experience of symptoms and incidents of illness?

The social consequences of superior female longevity are to some extent quite obvious, yet more investigation of them seems to be needed. An imbalance of males and females means that some women will be unable to form families; this raises interesting questions about the occupational and recreational roles of the single woman, perhaps especially in the large cities where the United States' population is increasingly concentrated. Even more important are the very large numbers of widows who outlive their husbands. Most of these women have a relatively slight chance to remarry, and they face problems of loneliness, of economic insecurity, and often of trying to find useful social roles.

Race

Of all the inequalities in the distribution of health—and life—chances in American society, the most striking are those that accompany the general inequality between racial groups. Although Negroes have benefited from the overall decline in population mortality, they continue to be at a disadvantage in virtually every category of death and illness. Negro health deficits begin early and continue at all ages up to seventy-five; prenatal and infant mortality are substantially higher for Negroes. The clustering of disadvantage among nonwhites is evident at every hand. For example, infant mortality rates for central Harlem are two and one-half times as great as those for certain other New York City districts. Later in life, measures in the same community show the mortality rate for tuberculosis to be sixteen times higher in central Harlem than in the district where tuberculosis mortality is lowest. Consistently, nonwhite rates of disabling illness and of the chronic diseases are higher. The rates for hospitalized mental illness are also higher. The Negro homicide rate is seven times the white rate. Indeed, suicide is virtually the only significant cause of death that finds white risks exceeding Negro risks. By any measure, then, the general health patterns of Negroes are poorer than those of whites.

Thus the penalties of lower caste membership in the United States are vividly expressed in the field of health. To all the other burdens of social inferiority must be added the threat of illness and the shortening of life. It has been remarked that health is a chief "enabling resource" for the individual in a competitive society that places heavy emphasis on skillful and efficient personal functioning. This means that those who lack health are without basic equipment to compete in life, to achieve desirable jobs, and to expend the energy necessary for self-fulfillment. Along with educational deficiencies, health risks serve to compound Negro disadvantages across the board. One might say that Negroes face not only a defective, foreshortened structure of opportunities but that they also have an unfavorable base of the individual competence essential to seizing and exploiting opportunity. Inevitably, given the involvement of health with education, economics, and total style of living, second class citizenship entails second class health. Nowhere else in our society is the fact that health and illness are interdependent with the totality of human circumstance more convincingly and cruelly illustrated.

The roots of this shocking maldistribution of illness are apparent in bold outline but unquestionably complex in causal detail. Like those of the poor, the annals of the racially disfavored are neither short nor simple: they are lifelong configurations of hazard and are incredibly tangled, snarled in a capricious social fate. Broadly speaking, the Negro suffers from lack of access to the conditions that are thought to promote *good* health and a corresponding lack of access to the facilities of care that might cushion and alleviate *ill* health. And the impact of these closed doors is probably heightened by the psychological strain that imbues the life of the underdog, the personal vigilance and diminished self-esteem that are the price of inferiority long maintained.

Negro disadvantage in health-promoting factors begins with poor maternal care. Negro women are much less likely to enjoy prenatal care, and if they do obtain it they do so later in pregnancy. Hence, the danger of birth complications resulting from poor nutrition, physiological difficulties, and injury to the mother is markedly raised. The conditions of birth itself are more hazardous because many more nonwhite babies are born either outside the hospital with inadequate medical attention or in hospitals that are less well-staffed and equipped than those available to white mothers. In early life the conditions of the family environment are more likely to include crowding, poor hygiene, malnutrition, and a host of other potentially deleterious features. Later in the life arc the Negroes' path is likely to be distinguished not only by the continuation (and accumulation) of all these deficits but also by an inferior schooling that generates cognitive incompetence and an inferior job entailing the negative results of dull, dangerous, or dirty work. Ghettoes and rural slums encourage impulse release in interpersonal violence and in the health-threatening indulgence of drug or alcohol excess.

Throughout their life span nonwhites typically obtain poorer health care than whites. Among the reasons for inadequate care are discrimination, economic disability, and very importantly, lack of initiative and responsiveness in the client group itself. That is, facilities are poorer to begin with and the consumers of health care are not well prepared to use extant resources. They are often called the "hard-to-reach." Their conceptions of illness and what might be done about it are radically different from those cherished by public health professionals. In addition, as we saw in Chapter 2, the helping relationship is likely to be flawed by disparate expectations on the part of treater and treated, so that any therapeutic effort is weakened by difficulties of interpersonal style. The distribution of health between the races is, then, an index to causal and therapeutic concerns. It is also, more broadly, an index to the immense social failure that punctuates the American dream of equality with recurrent nightmares.

Socioeconomic Rank

It is no accident that most of the uneven occurrence of health between races is repeated when we consider the distribution of health among socioeconomic groups in modern society. On nearly every count, membership in the lower socioeconomic layers carries health penalties similar to those exacted of Negroes. Most studies, indeed, demonstrate that social class disadvantage is intrinsically more significant than color as such. Poor Negro health states may be largely accounted for by the highly probable coincidence of being both a Negro and a member of the lower class. That is, the health of middle class Negroes more nearly resembles that of middle class whites than that of the economically deprived of either race. Hence, we are driven to the master conclusion that the pattern of disadvantage is circular, and cumulative: being at the bottom of the social ranking generates a host of disabilities. These disabilities, in turn, sap the intelligence, energy, and physical tone that are required to move out of the lowest positions.

Evidence for the differential distribution of illness by social class is varied and convincing. Overwhelmingly, of course, the associations are inverse—the lower the social ranking, the higher the risk of ill health. But the exceptions to this general rule are also worthy of note. An especially interesting exception is found in coronary heart disease, where we are forced to reverse the usual line of questioning: not, What social disadvantages promote ill health? but in a real sense, What "advantages" expose the affluent and achieving male to heightened risk? The life styles of executive and professional occupations are increasingly the object of intense study; one might conceive of them as the causal microcosm, the individual and familial expressions of those broader currents of urbanization-industrialization rehearsed earlier. Heightened risks of illness and death in these "exceptional" contexts, where risk is directly rather than inversely correlated with social ranking, also provoke curiosity about the processes of self-selection. There may be significant patterns of personality characteristics that predispose their bearers both to successful careers of occupational attainment *and* to special vulnerability to complex social psychological agents of disease.

Many of the data supporting the links between social rank and illness are found in differential rates of illness among occupational groups. This is because such data are relatively easy to obtain and because in industrial societies occupation is the most accurate single indicator of general social standing. Studies of gross occupational clusters, such as U.S. census categories, and studies in large firms with diversified labor forces point again and again to increasing rates of illness as one descends the occupational ladder. The differences go far beyond the expectable distinctions that would be attributable to the heightened exposure to accidents, toxic substances, weather, and the like, typical of lower status jobs. Incidence of infectious diseases, absences from work, and level of subjective reporting of symptoms all pile up in the less well-rewarded and less prestigious occupations. The portrait for the United States is roughly repeated by evidence from Great Britain: long-term records for England and Wales, for example, show symmetrical relations between illness and mortality rates and occupational ranking. Again, as in the racial contrasts in the United States, we discover a clustering of disadvantage. The view from the bottom is not limited to deprivation of money, possessions, and status but, instead, deprivations ramify to entail decreased chances for health and for life itself.

Another vital area of social class differences in illness is the mental diseases. Repeated investigations have shown a higher prevalence of severe mental illness, especially the schizophrenic psychoses, in the lowest socioeconomic groups. (Although certain psychoses are not distributed in such a skewed fashion and a few investigators have found reversals of the general trend, schizophrenia is much the most common diagnostic category and thus accounts for numerical preponderance among the disadvantaged.) To the distinctions in illness rates must be added still greater discrepancies among social classes in length of hospitalization and outlook for recovery. Not only do the most disadvantaged groups show a heightened risk of psychological disturbance but also, once the disturbance has occurred, members of these groups are likely to receive less-favored types of treatment, a longer hospital stay, and a lessened possibility of a return to full social functioning.

Two factors underline the potential importance of social psychological research to an understanding of the uneven distribution of mental health in populations. The first is the presumably very complicated network of cause in which conventional organic aspects are of unknown weight for most varieties of disease. The second is the character of psychological "dis-ease" itself, its manifestation in deranged patterns of interpersonal functioning rather than in physical symptomatology. (Overt physiological upset, such as sweating palms, shallow breathing, insomnia, and rapid heart beat, is an exceedingly useful indicator of psychological disease. However, the expression of disturbance that leads to the individual's being judged ill by others, and most often by himself, is not characteristically a physical incapacity but a rupture in the performance of social roles and in the person's confident sense of selfhood.)

Psychiatric epidemiology is now moving beyond the identification of social class differences in illness and treatment, toward a specification of the total social environment that precipitates or cushions psychological upset. Some of the most promising effort in this vein is the work of Alexander H. and Dorothea Leighton and their colleagues in a maritime province of Canada. Here, the evidence tentatively points toward differences in the distribution of illness according to the organized or disorganized fabric of community life. Psychiatric symptoms are found to be at a higher level in the populations of "disorganized" communities (those marked by economic insufficiency, weak leadership, confused values, and interpersonal hostility) than in those of seemingly better integrated locales.

Mental retardation, especially as measured by level of cognitive performance in school settings, is still another chronic illness that shows very dramatic differences in distribution. "Mild" mental retardation is by far the largest category. This disability is not ordinarily discovered until the child is exposed to the demands of formal education, where he slips steadily behind the level of intellectual competence displayed by his classmates. Mild retardation is a marginal illness that is thought to depend heavily on the kinds of stimulation offered the growing child and on the way others perceive his capabilities. Important evidence indicates that changes in the learning situation may not only induce substantial competence in the retarded child but may also bring about something like a reversal or retrieval of the mild condition. The prevalence of mild retardation follows the configuration sketched above for most illnesses, including psychological disorder. That is, the economically disadvantaged and culturally deprived sectors of the population are strikingly overrepresented among the mildly retarded. Thus we are led once more by uneven rates of disorder to question the possible range of causal factors and to search out elements in the life styles of different groups that may predispose to exaggerated or diminished risk.

Summary

Only when we know where major health problems reside in populations can we begin to assess the multitude of potential antecedents of illness. The selected instances of discrepant rates touched upon in this chapter lead quite naturally into a quest for explanation. We wish to know what it is that accounts for glaring differences in the mortality and morbidity experiences of various groups. We also wish to know the roots of discrepant experiences in the prevention and treatment of illness. Chapters 7 and 8 will address themselves to these sorts of issues. *What* is it about urbanization-industrialization that makes chronic degenerative diseases flourish, while stifling the infectious diseases? *How* is sexual identity or stage in the life cycle related to varied risks? *Why* should disprivileged racial or socioeconomic group membership expose the individual to lessened chances for long life and good health?

CHAPTER 7

Social Epidemiology:
The Search for Cause

Contemporary approaches favor a multicausal and processual model of the way an individual stays well or becomes ill. The attack is multicausal because the health states of most compelling interest appear to rest on a concatenation of biological vulnerability, psychological dynamics, and social situational expectations. It is processual because we do not conceive of illness as a single event that impinges on a stationary organism but, instead, as a sequence of malfunctioning phased in and out with the exigencies of experience as individuals and families move along the arc of life. The current thrust of social epidemiology may be phrased as an effort to assess the links between the life styles of populations—their total configuration of actions and reactions in social time and space—and the health risks to which those populations are vulnerable. In this thrust, investigators clearly require a conceptual model of causation that goes beyond the germ theory of disease, that pays as much attention to social and psychological agents as to microorganisms. The older medical rhetoric—What's he got and what's good for it?—is giving way to a much more complicated question, or series of questions, that might be put thus: What is it about his way of life that cushions or exacerbates certain health risks, and how may he be helped to live with the burden of chronicity?

Cause and Linked Systems

One avenue to an understanding of the multidetermined nature of illness may be found in the model of "linked open systems," as first presented by biologist Ludwig von Bertalanffy and elaborated by William Caudill for social medicine. Essentially, this model contends that living systems are invariably hooked together and mutually permeable, influencing one another in a welter of cause-and-effect relationships. Events occuring in one sphere of these linked human processual systems cannot be confined to that sphere alone but ramify in their impacts upon adjoining spheres. For example, a psychological event, such as a thwarted need for affection, not only influences the personality system of the individual but also is very likely to bear consequences for his biological system and his capacity to act effectively as a member of a network of interpersonal relations. Causes and effects cannot be contained within the system that appears to be their primary locus, but they branch out into all those life processes in which the individual is engaged. Many illustrations of these patterns are familiar, as when a biological event, say the onset of diabetes, spills over into the person's concept of himself and his relations with members of his family, or when a social event, say the loss of a loved other, takes hold upon the psychological system through grief and upon the organic system through insomnia. Perhaps the most convincing sort of evidence for this systemic interplay, this demonstration that groups of systems or the whole life-space become ill or well, is seen in the "clustering" of illnesses among certain individuals and family units. Both disease symptoms and episodes of illness pile up in a nonrandom fashion, so that the ill person tends to become ill in a variety of ways and the family with a problem tends to become a "multiproblem" family. Health and illness proliferate in living systems, feeding upon themselves, so to speak.

It is probably more accurate to say that the epidemiologist searches for causes of illness, for linked chains of influence, than that he seeks *a* cause. We are beginning to believe that what counts in generating a given state of health is not a solitary causal villain but a *configuration of disposing elements*. Although his method of investigation, suspicion, and elimination resembles the techniques of the fictional detective hero, the researcher does not commonly uncover a murderer of life or a thief of comfort, but he uncovers a series of implicated factors. The idea that a configuration of elements underlies many states of ill health may be pointed up by the presumed etiology of tuberculosis. Tuberculosis also illustrates the interpenetration of biological and social psychological systems. We know that the tubercle bacillus is harbored by very large numbers of the population and yet that only a small fraction of these persons possessing the causal microorganism ever develop frank symptomatology of the disease "tuberculosis." Hence, it becomes necessary to identify "what else" is involved, what other life processes serve either to protect the individual from the full-blown illness or to encourage the development of symptoms.

Knowledge of the full configuration is far from complete, but the inquiries of Thomas H. Holmes and his associates have begun to establish certain quite interesting patterns. Plotting the distribution of tuberculosis in Seattle, they found high concentrations among men living alone in the central city. Further study of men hospitalized with tuberculosis showed the disease to be associated with alcoholism, divorce, and very importantly, the relatively recent experience of stressful life events, such as separation from a close relative or loss of a job. Another clue lay in the disproportionately frequent occurrence of the disease among individuals who were isolated from the main body of their fellows through residence in sections of the city populated mainly by other groups than their own, for example, Negroes living in predominantly white suburbs. Altogether, these and allied investigations have begun to reveal that the effect of the "causal germ" in tuberculosis is highly dependent on a variety of other circumstances in which the individual is enmeshed. Apparently the development of the full-blown disease is encouraged by the kinds of life experience that wrench the person away from his accustomed interpersonal environment, that expose him to the social stress of isolation and, probably, to a corresponding degradation or disarray in his self-image.

Indeed, the example of tuberculosis may be multiplied in a

number of health states that are associated with separation or isolation of the individual. For the bulk of illnesses, notably including mental illness, the separated, divorced, widowed, and single population is at heightened risk in comparison with members of intact family units. This repeated observation has not thus far been supplemented either by intensive research or by a coherent framework of theoretical explanation. It seems reasonable to assume that membership in a family group is in certain ways protective of good health: two distinct possibilities are that the network of interpersonal ties in a family involves some degree of mutual watchfulness, of concern for one another's health processes, and that the sense of self is reinforced by the stimulus of affectionate others. Correlatively, one would anticipate that the single individual is deprived of such supports. Obviously, too, in the case of the divorced and never-married there may be predisposing personality factors that militate against enduring family relationships and also contribute to an added health risk.

Family membership, however, is not an unmixed health blessing. The levels of wellness in families exhibit a systemic character, such that family health seems to be more than a summing-up of the conditions of each member. Apart from genetic sharing of disabilities among relatives and the increased exposure to infection stemming from life at close quarters, some familial styles of behavior seem to promote the clustering of illness. For example, in studies of families of the chronically disabled, the risks that some member *other* than the first-identified "case" will also be disabled or frequently ill are shown to be significantly increased. It may be that the task of nurturing one ill member constitutes extra exposure for the remaining members. Perhaps more tantalizing is the possibility that dispositions toward certain types of "dis-ease" are in fact "communicated" through interpersonal influence, that relatives learn from one another how to adopt favored versions of illness and wellness. In the psychological illnesses, especially, there is impressive, if scattered, evidence that neurotic stylings of behavior may be taught and shared. Quite apart from the rare, extreme instances of shared delusion (folie à deux), some family histories show repetitive patterns of maladaptive response.

Cause and Group Membership

If differential rates of illness in family groups indicate that the social relationships within this tightly knit system may be etiologically significant, what may be said of the many other group memberships that contribute to the person's identity? Chief among the social involvements that are provocatively linked to health are *race, social class, occupation,* and *community of residence.* Another type of membership frequently related to health chances is more subtle: it concerns the *extent to which the individual is exposed to rapid change in his life circumstances or the extent to which the various segments of his experience hang together in a meaningful way.*

In Chapter 6, we discussed certain features of racial group membership that appear to dispose the person toward good or ill health. As noted, to a considerable extent these features of the condition of "being nonwhite" overlapped with the characteristics of "being lower social class," whatever one's race. Now we may propose that the etiology of various states of ill health in the most disadvantaged sectors of the population rests not only on the obvious defects of nutrition, housing, preventive medical care, and so on, but also on a syndrome of social psychological insufficiency. This syndrome may be visualized to consist of two main parts: *generalized inferiority feelings,* a defect in the self-picture, and *generalized incompetence,* a defect in the trained capacity to function in the rewarded social roles of American society. Given a diminished image of the self, a tentative assumption of unworthiness, the underdog in our society finds the image confirmed by cumulative experiences of failure in those contexts that seem to matter most to upholders of dominant middle class values. A damaged sense of identity and a damaged sense of competence may themselves be viewed as intrinsic "diseases" of the total psychosocial equilibrium of the individual. In turn, these deficits may provide a necessary, if not sufficient, causal strand in the production of a range of illnesses.

A careless and uncertain regard for the self—indeed, the absence of any conviction of significant selfhood—would appear to be the almost inevitable result of those early deprivations undergone in family, school, and neighborhood by lower class Negroes and whites. Parents, themselves socially scorned, cannot but transmit feelings of worthlessness to the child. Schools, geared to the culture of middle class aspirants for the conventional prizes of our society, reinforce the underdog child's premonitions of inadequacy. The community at large treats its disadvantaged population with a contempt seldom veiled and, if then, only muffled in a cloak of patronizing exhortation. Psychiatrists Abram Kardiner and Lionel Ovesey have termed the destruction of self-regard and the creation of self-hate the Negro's "mark of oppression," a caste stigma borne not on the forehead but in the vitals. Everything considered, it seems reasonable to think that this mark is not confined to Negroes, although it is probably accentuated among them; the economically and socially disprivileged of whatever color bear the mark of inferiority. All that we know about the pervasive nature of health and illness leads us to postulate that a defective self-picture, a weak and blurred adumbration of who one is and for what one counts, is integral to the susceptibility to illness.

Generalized incompetence is clearly related to the feeling of inferiority. The weak ego, and often the confused identity, of the oppressed child does not provide the motivational springs for achieving tasks. An unsure self cannot be consistently assertive, cannot assume the masterful stance toward physical and social environment that seems to underlie the growth of competence. The investigations of clinical psychologist Robert W. White and others into the development of "competence motivation" in the child indicate that early in his life the child must learn a posture of manipulative mastery, of free play with an environment responsive to his efforts. This early thrust toward effective coping is then necessarily supplemented by two important chains of events: symbolic stimulation in the household, with the parents as key agents, and continued stimulation and reward in the school, with teachers and peers as key agents. There must be a diet of words, colors, objects, processes, and sounds rich enough to induct the child into that symbolic universe that constitutes the "real world" of inhabitants of an advanced industrial society like the contemporary United States.

The disadvantaged child, white or Negro, commonly enjoys only a foreshortened structure of opportunities for the development of competence motivation. Like inferiority, incompetence is cumulative. Lacking a sufficient early symbolic input, the children of poverty and discrimination begin formal schooling under a grave handicap and then find their incompetent performances reinforced by classroom failure and subsequent job failure. Burdened with successive experiences of failure and lacking an inner conviction of fundamental worth, the individual is less likely to exhibit healthy patterns of living. The core "dis-ease" in living and functioning comfortably with self and others is then expressed in varieties of ill health. Mild mental retardation and mental illness are the most apparent illness outcomes; they also possess the greatest face validity as logical results of the syndrome of social psychological insufficiency. It is quite unlikely, however, that functional mental disturbance is the sole health consequence of this syndrome. Inferiority and incompetence breed more of the same; they proliferate in the individual life space. Hence, our assumptions about multiple causality and linked open systems in human affairs persuade us that inadequate management of the self can ramify in the organic system, and in health behavior generally, to contribute substantially to the uneven gradient of risk over a broad spectrum of ill health states.

Differences in the distribution of illness among occupational groups tend, as we have noted, to recapitulate the inverse relation between social rank and illness. Although by no means true of all "dis-eases," occupational rank is, in general, negatively associated with health risk: the lower the occupation is ranked, the higher the illness rates exhibited by its members. This is, of course, the picture we should expect in view of the close connection among race, social class, and attainment in the world of work. But if generalized felt inferiority and generalized incompetence are implicated in the less sure grasp on health that workers at lower job levels show—and they do seem germane to phenomena as separate as accidents, absence from work, and total reported symptoms of sickness—what *protective* mechanisms may be operating to preserve the health of the highly ranked?

One interesting epidemiological clue to the association of high occupational status and good health may be found in the central value attributed to work in Western industrialized societies. This is the arena where the male (and increasingly, the female) demonstrates a major share of his social competence and gains a major share of his rewards from others. Work has, indeed, been elevated to such an important pitch that job performance assumes a moral tone; regular occupational contributions come to serve as a validation of the self. Unemployed men during the depression of the 1930s in the United States illustrated the point vividly: as significant as their loss of income was their loss of self-esteem and the loss of esteem from those nearest them. If the job is central, if the individual's commitment to it is such that it makes up an absorbing activity, and if a fair measure of success has been achieved, we seem to have almost a countersyndrome to that social psychological insufficiency hypothesized above. A "syndrome of sufficiency," one might say, serves to enhance the person's healthy processes and to keep him robustly viable as a social actor. In large firms, executives, managers, and professionals are less often absent and manifest fewer felt symptoms than do employees at other levels. Thoroughly engaged and highly rewarded, they apparently enjoy a zest for life that is health-promoting.

Aspects of Stress

There is, then, ample evidence from the study of families, races, social classes, and occupations that sets of factors in the social experience of the person are significantly involved in his health. For fuller understanding of social etiology, it is appropriate to introduce the concept of *stress* and to try to link this idea to the manner in which health changes accompany life changes. Although there is no precise, widely accepted definition of this concept, observers are generally agreed that it consists of the interaction between a force external to the individual and his interpretation of or reaction to this force as expressed in discomfort he feels or in apparent symptoms. Thus a stressful event is one that impinges on the person in such a way as to call forth some change, conscious or unconscious, in his customary mode of bodily maintenance or psychological ease. We are here interested in a particular variety of stress that occurs in the social psychological universe and threatens the person's total security system in some way. The avenues of threat are, of course, legion, ranging from interference with basic human needs to disruptions in the self-picture and derangements in his accustomed pattern of social relatedness. Clearly, a good deal of our previous discussion centering on the deleterious effects of being isolated, being an underdog, and being unfulfilled in the work life is relevant to the problem of stress.

Numerous clinical studies, especially those falling under the inexact but useful heading of "psychosomatic medicine," afford dramatically convincing evidence that perceived threats to the self may be readily translated into a panoply of physiological expressions. There is also a well-established body of experimental data that shows how discomfort in social relations and its attendant psychological upsets finds ready outlets in the language of bodily signs. Thus an individual who is threatened with a blow to his forearm may exhibit on that arm the reddened weal consequent to being struck even when the blow does *not* physically take place; the person who is feeling disappointed or agitated about some life event may show the literal signs of anger in changes in the appearance of his stomach; patient and physician in psychotherapy record similar pulse rates accompanying the tenor of their interaction. We are concerned, however, with extending this type of linkage beyond the single case history, with assessing the consistencies and differences of stress among population groups undergoing diverse patterns of life experience.

Lawrence E. Hinkle, Jr., and Harold G. Wolff, among others, have found a general relationship between the vicissitudes of living and the rates of illness. By following several groups of men and women over a period of years, they have been able to demonstrate that individual styles of falling ill or staying healthy rest on the person's perception of his life situation. As Hinkle and Wolff conclude:

> good health among our informants was the result not of a generally superior adaptive capacity but rather of their having existed in a life situation which satisfied their own peculiar needs and aspirations, however these might differ from those of the population in general. Conversely, we infer that ill health may be evidence of poor adaptive capacity but is not necessarily so; it appears to occur when an individual exists in a life situation which places demands upon him that are excessive in terms of his ability to meet them or which fails to satisfy his own peculiar needs and aspirations.[1]

[1] Lawrence E. Hinkle, Jr., and Harold G. Wolff, "Health and the

These investigators noted similar clusterings of illness among American men and women employed in different jobs, as well as among a sample of Chinese immigrants to the United States. Those who felt the pressure of adverse circumstances or who found their work experiences jarringly at odds with their aspirations showed illness rates much higher than their counterparts for a whole battery of diseases, ranging from upper respiratory episodes to anxiety and depression. The basic point, driven home again and again, is that illness experience in the large is significantly associated with total ways of living and total structures of personality. If we wish to understand the distribution of ill health in populations, we must attend not only to the conventional hazards of physical environments and microorganisms but also to those social relations and psychological characteristics that permeate the life history.

Social epidemiology customarily begins its search for cause by seeking out the sorts of distinctions in group experience identified thus far. Research may, however, start with the personality patterns of group members and try to determine how the individual's learned modes of functioning bring him into confrontation with a social milieu and, in turn, with varying health risks. A recent pertinent illustration of this strategy is the work of Meyer Friedman and Ray Rosenman, heart disease specialists, and clinical psychologist C. David Jenkins. These investigators initially noticed that, among a series of patients in their clinical practice, certain men seemed to be distinctively at risk of heart disease. Such individuals showed a repetitive clustering of behavior that marked a "coronary-prone" personality. They had a high drive for occupational achievement, haste, impatience, a strict, tense, energetic outpouring of resources directed to meeting deadlines and managing the pressures of the job. They were dedicated, vigilant men, acutely responsive to the demanding stimuli of an upper-middle class American life style. At length, the researchers succeeded in identifying what they termed "Type A" and "Type B" personalities. They followed large samples of men for several years and were able to distinguish the "A" individuals, just described, from "B" individuals, who were calmer, more easygoing,

Social Environment: Experimental Investigations," in Alexander H. Leighton, John A. Clausen, and Robert N. Wilson (eds.), *Explorations in Social Psychiatry* (New York: Basic Books, 1957), p. 131.

and less inclined to invest themselves so wholly in a pattern of striving. The "A" men, in turn, were found to experience significantly heightened risk of coronary heart disease. An urgent need for future research would seem to be to explore a variety of occupational and other social settings in which the two personality types are enmeshed, and to try to assess the contributions of personal characteristics as compared to social relational demands. Perhaps "A" individuals are self-selected for stressful jobs. At the same time, one might guess that, given a personality predisposition that increases the risk of illness, certain "cushions" in the realm of social interaction might serve partially to counteract the danger.

Social Change and Health Risk

If we are led to suspect that the stress of life is an important causal agent in disease and that this stress is generated by an amalgam of situational pressures and individual characteristics, the next step clearly is to specify the particular kinds of life event and kinds of personalities that join to produce unusual risks of illness. The kind of life event most often singled out for attention in social epidemiology is the movement of individuals along the life arc in such a way as to promote imbalance or incongruity among the different regions of their experience. Radical changes and inconsistencies in life circumstances frequently seem to expose people to deleterious health changes.

At the beginning of this chapter, tuberculosis was cited as a disease that disproportionately often affects those who have suffered breaks in the fabric of social relatedness. A number of other illnesses have been associated with peoples' movements in geographical and social space. Some evidence suggests that migrants from state to state are at increased risk of severe mental illness. And discontinuities in social space have been related to health risks as diverse as arthritis and mental disorder. Social psychological incongruity is especially marked in the instance of persons whose different social characteristics do not hang together in an appropriate fashion. For example, the individual whose various statuses are "uncrystallized" may bear a special risk. The illustrative case would be the person of high economic rank who nonetheless shows a low level of educational attainment or vice versa. Another recent investigation by Hinkle adds to this strand of evidence: following the careers of executives in a large industry, he found that the risk of heart attack at an early age was greater for employees who lacked a college education than for those who enjoyed this background. Presumably, the individual who enters an executive role after college has been "trained" for that occupational level and can comfortably accept it, whereas his counterpart who gains a high-level position without college preparation is exposed to a greater change in expectations. One might speculate that the latter has in a very real sense achieved more, and more rapidly, and thereby pays a health price.

Populations in the world today are experiencing social change that is faster and more far-reaching than has ever previously been the case. This change is of several types, but its most general characteristic is the vast technological and organizational shift usually called "urbanization-industrialization." In the less developed nations, it may be designated as development or modernization. Pervasive social change affects the lives people can lead, and as a consequence, it has significant implications for their health.

We have already traced salient *direct* health changes associated with industrialization, chiefly the transition from communicable and infectious diseases to chronic diseases, and the lengthening of life expectancy. But there are also increasingly apparent *indirect* changes that appear to be connected to crucial alterations in styles of living under social transition. These alterations commonly provoke, on a broad scale, the kind of imbalance among values, expectations, and social statuses sketched above. When social change occurs, it commonly moves at differing rates among the sectors of the total societal system. For instance, a given technological innovation may alter the conditions of work much more rapidly than the family structure or the religious values of the affected population change. Or, individuals may migrate to a modern city in search of employment, bringing with them the now inappropriate habits and perceptions of a rural lifetime.

Scattered but compelling recent evidence suggests that the linked processes of urbanization-industrialization ("inurbation," to use the barbarous but compact term of one observer) may indeed carry deleterious health consequences, at least during the period of speediest transition. John C. Cassel and Herman A. Tyroler investigated the health of a population of working men in a small industrial city in western North Carolina, and they found the group at highest risk of illness to be what they called "first-generation" factory employees. These were men who were the first members of their families to move from rural mountain villages into the style of life of factory workers. The "factory disciplines" of timeclocks, routinized jobs, and a cash economy were drastic shifts from a rural pace geared to natural rhythms and bounded by the social network of village kin. Men of the first generation were absent from work more often and exhibited more episodes of a variety of illnesses. Second-generation men, whose fathers had sought industrial work, did not experience the same heightened risk. As a population, they had presumably had more time to adapt to urban styles.

Several other studies offer clues pointing in the same general direction. Cassel and Tyroler, again, found heightened rates of coronary heart disease among rural men who lived in rapidly urbanizing counties. Ralph C. Patrick, Jr., and Tyroler discovered an association between the risks of high blood pressure and degree of "modernity" in the villages inhabited by Papago Indians, who stem from a very traditional Indian culture. Similarly, epidemiologist Ricardo Cruz-Coke reported that Easter Islanders, having lived in a remote, traditional society, showed a marked rise in blood pressure when they emigrated to metropolitan Lima, on the Peruvian mainland.

The guiding hypothesis in these types of investigations is that transition from one style of life to another is a source of stressful experience. Researchers are acutely challenged, however, to determine with more specificity *what* it is about urbanization, or any other profound shift in circumstance, that may be causally implicated in the production of certain diseases. This lack of specificity, as well as a paucity of dynamic hypotheses to link social events to illness events, plagues the field of social epidemiology. We are, in much of our work, stuck at the level of *associations*—rather than causal relations—between characteristics of population experience and their corresponding states of health. Yet our present, inadequate grasp of social causation in the medical world does not imply that nothing can be done to alleviate this aspect of health problems. *Even without* precise information about pathogenic agents in the modernization process, ways may be found to ease the passage from rural to urban life ways. *Even without* exact knowledge about why poverty and low social status are disproportionately the seedbeds of severe mental illness, much can be done to break the truly vicious circle of disadvantage.

In Chapter 8, we shall examine the other major thread of social medicine: the attempt to "treat" populations and communities by preventive and therapeutic strategies, involving especially an assessment of why people do or do not respond to professionals' helping overtures.

Social Epidemiology:
Patterns of Treatment

All the issues analyzed in Chapters 1 through 7 converge at length upon a single complex goal: bettering the states of health and, by direct implication, the quality of life of populations. The quest for higher levels of wellness in large groups represents a summing-up and point of application for knowledge as diverse as the definition of health, the nature of the helping relationship, the institutional structure of modern health care, and the distribution and causal underpinning of disease. Population treatment constitutes a vast field of endeavor for the student of medicine and society—a field that has thus far been cultivated only in the most scattered and superficial fashion.

Bases of Treatment

To say that our understanding of healthy and ill processes in human living is less than adequate is a trite, flat announcement. It is also perfectly true. We are plagued with acute problems of conceptualization and measurement at every turn. When the social and psychological factors affecting health are at issue, it is exceedingly difficult to reach agreement on the definition of "social class" or "occupational mobility" or "stress." When the resultant state of health is at issue, it is equally hard to find consensus about what constitutes "mental illness" or "hypertension." A major obstacle to more precise understanding is surely composed of the very habits of mind we bring to the health enterprise: we are schooled to look for a solidity and clarity in our categories that probably do not exist in the nature of living things. Most of the targets of interest are processual continua, marked by fine shadings of difference rather than bold, distinctive "breaks" among categories. This is obviously the case with social psychological antecedents, such as role behavior or personality structure. It is very probably the case with the bulk of chronic illnesses, where the question is not so much, Has he got it, or not? but, How much does he have, and how does it affect his competence as a social actor?

Nevertheless, the contemporary health sciences have garnered a good deal more sophistication than they have been able to put to use. In the United States, especially, the gulf between technical medical elegance and the level of care actually provided is shockingly wide. Infant mortality is a familiar example. History's most affluent and medically expert nation, the United States, lags behind many other less handsomely endowed countries in its ability to keep babies alive. Some of the reasons for our relatively feeble capacity to apply a high quality of health care were underlined in Part One of this book: barriers to patient-practitioner interaction; the numbers and preparation of health professionals; and the haphazard organization of medical facilities, abetted by a narrow, fragmented approach to community organization. Joined with these failings is an insufficient effort at comprehensive and scientifically rigorous planning to initiate and assess health programs.

The treatment of populations, whether focused on early intervention to ward off disease or on therapeutic strategies to manage an existing level of illness, is commonly deficient in two major respects. First are failures to pose an accurate statement of the health problem, the measures to be undertaken to meet it, and the goals of the program instituted by health professionals. That is, we do not usually exhibit enough awareness or depth in our conception of precisely what we are doing; we do not ask clearly, for example, why we mount a tuberculosis control program, exactly what the components, in action, shall be, and what magnitude of change in the occurrence or virulence of tuberculosis is being sought by these means. Second, the proponents of health programs too seldom question the actual value or outcome of their chosen strategies. A blind faith in the efficacy of activity, a faith well-rooted in the characteristic American passion for doing and busyness, replaces a serious scheme for assessing outcomes. Yet a program of treatment that is not evaluated promises little cumulative effect. Not only do the true results of the program remain hidden, but there is also little chance of generalizing the experience to similar health problems in other community contexts. In part, the neglect of shrewd evaluation rests on the difficulty of defining program goals and of measuring them once defined. Too often, the obvious and easily measured indicator of treatment efforts (such as the number of contacts between health professionals and a target group) is regarded as an end in itself, as an ample gauge of a program's efficacy, and neglects the important and usually more subtle indicators (such as a shift in the health level of the population).

Treatment or prevention begins with a series of strategic decisions about who to treat, how and why the target population is to be approached, and who the agents of the program are to be. No program can really be more effective than the quality of the defining or presenting data will permit. Any plan, that is, must be founded upon an adequate baseline of the facts of life as revealed in epidemiological surveys of health states and social surveys of the characteristics of the target. Then, both the current levels of health and the nature of the population at risk must be seen as embedded in a texture of the prevailing culture: the values, habits, and forms of social relatedness that will make up the scene of any proposed health action. The most precise possible data concerning the distribution of illness must be articulated with a profile of community organization, such as that suggested in Chapter 5.

Given the relative scarcity of health manpower and facilities, it is obvious that all versions of the desirable cannot be entertained simultaneously. Only accurate epidemiological knowledge, complemented by insight into the way of life of the population, can afford a basis for setting priorities of treatment.

Presumably, any given pattern of attack on illness is precipitated by a configuration of decisions. Some of these decisions occur by fiat, in that a particular health professional or governmental policy maker decides more or less arbitrarily that a certain program is necessary; some take place following an informed weighing and balancing of mortality or morbidity rates; increasingly often, some program decisions are also taken in consultation with the target group, paying attention to their own *perceived* health needs as well as to the medical agent's diagnosis of the situation. Unfortunately, many programs planned via the first route, that of fiat, owe their creation less to either objectively measured or subjectively felt health problems than to the heavy hand of tradition. They are customary, regarded as "always needed," and routinely applied with scant reference to the current, pressing issues affecting *this* particular population.

Priorities

Fixing priorities in the treatment of the community-as-patient may well be the most complex and significant task for the public health worker and for other varieties of medical personnel. The process calls into question a range of factors in addition to the "purely medical," notably the realities of social power and cultural values. Ozzie Simmons, social anthropologist, has drawn attention to an especially striking instance of the way in which socioeconomic discrepancies may distort the allocation of health resources. Before the development of effective immunization, huge amounts of money and publicity were centered on the effort to cope with poliomyelitis, a dread disease but one of comparatively low incidence. These resources were greater than those devoted to tuberculosis, a more "familiar" disease but one of comparatively high incidence. Yet there was a revealing difference in the segments of the nation's population at highest risk of these two disabilities: polio attacked the advantaged middle class group more frequently, whereas tuberculosis was primarily concentrated among the poor, the politically and socially powerless.

Cultural values, especially as evidenced in beliefs about the nature of health and about the varying dramatic valences attached to diverse types of illness, importantly influence the alternatives of treatment. A well-known illustration is found in attempts to fluoridate community water supplies. Here, the medical rationale for health action is clear-cut. Fluoridation is safe, effective, and cheap. It should presumably receive a high and unambiguous priority in local programing. Yet, because a plethora of ideological factors came to cluster around fluoridation efforts, from fear of contamination to a fear of political plotting or an argument that civil rights were endangered, many cities' fluoridation programs were deflected or stillborn.

Because overt disease is a more compelling spur to health action than is the absence of vitality or the foreshortening of achievement, direct therapy often takes precedence over preventive or enhancing programs. An emphasis on curing disease rather than on promoting health affects priorities in many areas. The disproportion is exemplified in mental retardation. Although the great bulk of "mild" mental retardation has no identified organic cause and is believed to have its roots at least partially in early social deprivations, the major proportion of medical resources is directed toward the quite rare caseload of severe and profound mental retardates. These seriously disabled individuals, especially if their condition can be clearly related to genetic defect or brain injury, consume the attention of health professionals and the chief supplies of money and equipment. At the same time, a relatively small fraction of health program effort is devoted to research and amelioration among the quite large marginal population the members of whom are functionally impaired. A mongoloid child or hydrocephalic idiot is more compelling than the slow learner who drops steadily behind his classmates.

Another instance of priority setting that illustrates both social power factors and the way that treatment overshadows prevention may be seen in the distribution of health resources among the child population and the adult and aged population. Children do not vote, nor do their potential abilities and disabilities strike the eye as forcefully as the diminished physical state of the old. Dispassionately, one would have to assume that a nation's investment in fostering competent functioning among children has a much greater payoff than does the cushioning of impairment among the elderly. Yet both political prudence and cultural values dictated that medicare in the United States should precede comprehensive health services to children.

In effect, the assignment of priorities in medical programs hinges on the considerations reviewed in Chapter 1. If we define health merely as the absence of overt symptoms, then it is the symptoms of illness that must absorb health resources. If young people as a population and prevention as a strategy are to gain a high priority, the society must entertain some concept of *positive* health. Only then can the cultivation of competence be viewed as seriously as we now view the repair of health deficits.

The Context of Care

Granted that certain priorities have been set, that the health of a target group has been assessed and a program has been tentatively designed to alter the prevailing health conditions for the better, the social epidemiologist contends that a further vital kind of information is needed. Knowing what the primary health problems of a group are is not enough. Health is interlaced with the whole of social life and may not be ripped out of its context in the round of everyday behavior and beliefs. The gist of "what more" the program planner needs to know has been concisely expressed by Benjamin D. Paul:

> A celebrated malariologist who worked on the Panama Canal project made a remark which lingers in the memory of his public health disciples. "If you wish to control mosquitoes," he said, "you must learn to think like a mosquito." The cogency of this advice is evident. It applies, however, not only to mosquito populations one hopes to damage but also to human populations one hopes to benefit. If you wish to help a community improve its health, you must learn to think like the people of that community. Before asking a group of people to assume new health habits, it is wise to ascertain the existing habits, how these habits are linked to one another, what functions they perform, and what they mean to those who practice them.[1]

[1] Benjamin D. Paul, *Health, Culture and Community* (New York: Russell Sage Foundation, 1955), p. 1.

Of course, the health professional cannot know "everything" about a target group, and in a very real sense he can never know enough. But he must break loose from an easy assumption that the population to be helped is a uniform or standard aggregate of individuals who share exactly his own aims and theories about health and illness. At the very least, those who presume to prevent or treat require five orders of information:

1. *Culture:* What are the dominant values and beliefs that govern the group's outlook on the world? What are their ideals of proper conduct in recurrent life situations, of the social roles attached to different ages and sexes, and of preferred family, work, and community organization?
2. *Health ideas:* What concepts of health and sickness are most firmly held? Are certain illnesses feared because they are thought to involve moral or religious transgressions? Who is the customary source of knowledge about disease, and who is the usual therapist?
3. *Social structure:* How are people arrayed in family systems? Where and how do they work? How is the community divided by social and economic distinctions? What are the patterns of child raising that prepare individuals for life in this society?
4. *Community organization:* What are the political and economic institutions of the community? Who are the leaders in various phases of local activity? How are significant issues in public life usually resolved?
5. *Group membership:* With which groups do people identify? What are their formal and informal ties of association? How is their behavior conditioned by the style of life typical of their social class position?

Program Acceptance

Most treatment programs, and nearly all attempts to intervene in or to prevent illness, depend for effectiveness on the active collaboration of the target population. Hence, the question of program "acceptance" has become a significant concern of medical social investigation. Studies of population response to the tactics of health professionals have been mainly centered upon two sorts of group difference, that between Western and non-Western cultures and that between middle class and lower class subcultures within the United States. The root dilemma is the same in each instance: How can the medical professional, technically equipped to offer superior health services, appeal successfully to people who do not share his knowledge, his value system, or his immersion in the health enterprise? How, more-over, can lay respondents be convinced to make the changes in behavior implicit in most efforts to better health levels, particu-larly in those instances where the health risks are undramatic and not immediately apparent?

"Thinking like a mosquito" in public health demands that the analyst use his empathic talents to feel his way into the meaning of life situations in the group at risk. He must, that is, sensitively assess the way his respondents define the nature of the human interactions that will have to occur if a program is to be achieved. Above all, the proposed shift in behavior must be in-terpreted in a manner that makes sense in the respondent's life space, that connects itself to existing perceptions and habits. And the ancient injunction to the healer—that his ministrations do no harm—has to be expanded, so that the things not to be harmed include the integrity of the client's culture as well as the integrity of his body. A move toward improved health should not contra-vene other, deeply felt values. Indeed, it ordinarily stands little chance of doing so because health as an isolated end in itself does not often stand at the top of peoples' hierarchy of the desir-able or the necessary.

Of course, few health professionals would hazard a direct op-position to the population's entrenched ways of life, but contra-dictions are often implicit in a given program. Going against the grain of what the Victorian economist and social philosopher Walter Bagehot termed "the cake of custom" is usually the con-sequence of unintended side-effects and not a deliberate part of the medical approach. For example, when the cattle in a Near Eastern society were removed from the physical household in order to combat a fly-borne disease, the health workers were merely tackling a known source of germ transmission. They did not plan to disrupt domestic life and generate loneliness among housewives. Nevertheless, because cows in their customary place, a room next to the kitchen, had meant comfort and companionship to wives left alone all day, an important element of local culture had been inadvertently disrupted by the health innovation. Instances of this sort can be multiplied from accounts of Western scientific medicine's invading traditional societies.

A critical aspect of the effort to work with, rather than against, established routines of living lies in the choice of communicators and decision makers. In nearly every case, it has been found that the already prevailing channels of influence and centers of leadership are by far the most useful vehicles for promoting change. In non-Western cultures and lower social class groups in the West, communication and authority tend to be preeminently located in face-to-face relationships; influence is interpersonal and concrete. This implies that the authority of high-level officials and professional health workers is not usually a very potent source of innovation. Similarly, the reasoned health appeal embalmed in printed documents or broadcast via the mass media of communications may provoke the hoary question: Is anybody listening? Not only may sheer exposure to newspapers, pamphlets, and television be less, but the kind of attention given to formal discourse may be less exacting.

For the hard-to-reach sectors of the population, the so-called hard core of unresponsive individuals, special attempts to persuade usually involve the enlisting of local, natural leaders. If the accepted neighborhood or small-group leaders can be induced to push for acceptance of a health program, then their authority earned in other activities may be expected to carry over into health. The loudspeaker on the street or the face-to-face persuasions of neighbors are often more influential than are the more impersonal and formal communications channels.

In general, the person's accessibility to programs of prevention and treatment is directly related to his position in the hierarchy of local social life. The higher an individual's education and occupation, the more thoroughly imbedded he is in the flow of communal activity, the more responsive he is likely to be to the helping programs of health agents. Thus the more advantaged groups enjoy a favorable health outlook at both salients of epidemiological interest: their risks of most varieties of ill health are less, and their chances of being reached by prevention and therapy are greater. The evidence from a series of studies, notably illustrated in a sophisticated analysis of polio vaccine ac-

ceptance in Dade County, Florida,[2] shows convincing differences in responsiveness by social class. Of particular importance
in the Florida research was the level of participation in community life shown by the easily reached and the hard to reach.
Those who readily accepted a health program were both members of higher social class groups and members of a range of local
organizations. Furthermore, they had greater numbers of friends
and acquaintances and interacted with these associates more frequently. The hard to reach were educationally and occupation-
ally disadvantaged and were more isolated from the main currents of local concern; they reported fewer group memberships
and less frequent contact with friends. As the authors summed
up:

> In brief, this Non-Take [those who did not respond to the appeal
> to take polio vaccine] group, those with the poorest health protec-
> tion, were found also to be poor economically and educationally,
> poorly informed, poorly motivated, and poor in their interpersonal
> relations. The task of reaching them with health programs is a
> challenge.[3]

In the long run, health levels in a total society can probably
be best elevated by raising the social circumstances of disadvantaged bottom groups. That is, health can be improved by making
the underdog more nearly like the prosperous and the informed
and, hence, presumably, also rendering him at lessened risk and
heightened responsiveness to professional helpers. Part of this
general bettering process, too, would entail the associated fostering of a different system of values and personal postures toward
life's exigencies. Individuals of higher social rank in American
society exhibit those features of psychological make-up, especially the drives toward rational planning and mastery, that
typify the middle class health worker and constitute the ideal
image of a "good" client. But even assuming that such a transfor-
mation to homogeneity in health and related behavior were desirable, it clearly cannot be effected in the immediate future.

[2] Albert L. Johnson, C. David Jenkins, Ralph C. Patrick, Jr., and Travis
J. Northcutt, Jr., *Epidemiology of Polio Vaccine Acceptance*, Florida
State Board of Health Monograph 3 (1962).
[3] *Ibid.*, p. 82.

Therefore, ways must be found to bridge the subcultural gulf by means other than a radical restructuring of unresponsive clients.

Bridging Treater and Client

Several of these strategies have already been discussed, and their main burden would seem to be that health programs of whatever kind must be closely geared to the specific characteristics of different target groups. That is, the gulf must be initially bridged by energy and inventiveness on the part of health professionals. The treater of large populations can no more adopt a single, unitary model of health programing than the clinician can regard a series of individual patients as just alike in their needs and capabilities. Unfortunately, we are currently much more adept at diagnosing the clinical case than we are at shaping a social diagnosis for the health behavior of groups. As the Dade County researchers point out, a given health goal such as immunization must be pursued by alternate routes, by a number of subprograms especially tailored to the characteristics of recipient groups. If a newspaper campaign or discussions at civic clubs are effective with middle class respondents, then it must usually be complemented by block-by-block approaches using indigenous leaders with lower class respondents. The patient—the community—is not a solid entity; it is a complex system of relationships requiring exquisitely modulated pathways for bringing care to its various segments.

The epidemiology of program acceptance rests finally on both a firmer base of knowledge about clients and more alert, flexible behavior by health professionals. In Chapter 2, especially, we emphasized that the helping relationships are essentially to be seen as the junctures of social roles, the coming together of treater and treated. In this confrontation both parties are subject to change. It is more comfortable and professionally self-righteous to promote change in clients than to alter the health worker's own conventional perceptions and ways of doing things. Yet one might well maintain that a desperate need of our society is for greater sophistication and adaptiveness among the executive and professional cadres: a capacity for change among the agents of change themselves.

In *Man and Superman,* George Bernard Shaw suggested a rephrasing of the golden rule: "Do not do unto others as you would that they should do unto you; their tastes may not be the same." Just so, the first step in changing the health worker is perhaps to take this maxim seriously, to break him out of the ethnocentric habit of seeing his clients as mirror images of himself. Their aspirations, their ways of life, and particularly their conceptions of health and illness, may be vastly different. Yet it is, of course, not enough for the professional to substitute a "lower class" stereotype of the client for his former innocent conviction that each respondent shared his own devotion to rational health behavior. Rather, the agent of change must be encouraged not to harden and fix his image of client populations; he should be prepared to learn afresh, in swiftly moving situations, precisely what are the health needs and behavioral inclinations of *this* target group. Henry Major Tomlinson once remarked that "we see things not as they are, but as *we* are." Although the treater of populations has to school himself as far as possible to see things as they are, if he inevitably continues to look at the world largely through his own lens then this perceptual set should be one of maximum awareness and catholicity. The problem of the individual in a society like ours, with its supremely rapid pace of change, has been defined as that of "learning to learn." Health professionals must learn to learn about programs and populations. If they are trained only in "how to do it," their knowledge is soon hopelessly antique. In the words of former Secretary of Health, Education, and Welfare, John Gardner, the important yield of education is not how to do it, but "how to think about it."

CHAPTER 9

Health and Social Change:
The Health Future

Although Heraclitus observed long ago that "all is flux" and men have always known that change was the only constant in the human condition, change in our own era is marked by an acceleration and pervasiveness that set it qualitatively apart as social experience. Heraclitus used the image of the stream that could never be crossed twice in just the same manner because both the water and the individual crosser were subject to steady alteration. But today, the stream of change does not slip placidly by, instead, it rages like a torrent. Loren Eiseley gives dramatic expression to this changed character of change itself:

The long, slow turn of world-time as the geologist has known it, or the invisibly moving hour hand of evolution perceived only yesterday by the biologist, has given way in the human realm to a fantastically speeded-up social evolution induced by industrial technology. So fast does this change progress that a growing child strives to master the sociological mores of a culture which might, compared with the pace of past history, compress centuries of change into his lifetime. I, myself, like many among you, was born in an age which has already perished. At my death I will look my last upon a society which, save for some linguistic continuity, will seem increasingly alien and remote. It will be as though I peered upon my youth through misty centuries. . . . I will not be merely old: I will be a genuine fossil embedded in onrushing man-made time before my actual death.[1]

Social change is rapid because the speed with which techno-logical man can invent his own future has been so greatly in-creased by the numbers of innovators and the resources available to them. "Institutionalized innovation," a continuous habit of cre-ativity, has been built into industrial and scientific organization and, very notably, into contemporary medicine. Change is perva-sive because our tightly articulated society is so interdependent in its division of labor and so permeable to easy communication and transport. Moreover, the speed and scope of actual and po-tential change have induced a self-consciousness about the direc-tion in which the whole society or any of its subsystems is mov-ing. Thus change is increasingly often planned, deliberative, sought in the awareness of at least some of its consequences.

These characteristics of change have very apparent implica-tions for health, for medical institutions and professionals, and for the manifold relations between medicine and its environing society. Rapid shifts in the circumstances of life may generate certain risks to health; they may also, of course, act to enhance the possibilities of wellness. Transformations in technology imply transformations in social interaction, such that the organization of health care facilities and the roles of helping agents seem sure to change radically. Scientific mastery, within and without the medical domain, implies ever-greater control over certain human contingencies. Our vaunted capacity to manipulate ourselves and the world around us will probably mean that acceptable health levels will be more nearly taken for granted and more often held to be a routine right, a claim that all individuals can legitimately make on their society.

One drastic change that seems sure to affect medicine, that is indeed already shaping it, is the complex of developments usu-ally termed "automation." The ability to handle huge volumes of information in a systematic and readily repeatable fashion is profoundly influencing patterns of diagnosis, treatment, and re-search. Linked record systems make possible a new level of popu-

[1] Loren C. Eiseley, "The Freedom of the Juggernaut," *Mayo Clinic Proceedings*, 40 (1965), 7–21.

lation health surveillance, one in which fragments of the individual's health history can be meaningfully pieced together and group trends in illness processes can be observed. Automated systems aid diagnosis by rendering configurations of symptoms more speedily and comprehensively available; the computer can store knowledge and sift through alternatives much more powerfully than can a master clinician. The computer does not, of course, exhibit clinical intuition, a "feel" for appropriate diagnoses. Yet it can present the human agent of care with a map of possibilities, of alternatives upon which shrewd judgment can be more solidly grounded.

In treatment, automation enhances the precision of caretaking routines. Information control mechanisms can assure repeated exact drug dosage, and they are doing so today in some large hospitals. Automation importantly increases the scope of rational management in medical organizations, from the ordering of supplies to the prediction of bed vacancies. Further, such devices as closed-circuit television and electronic monitoring of physiological indicators contribute both to a close watchfulness on the patient's course and to a freeing of human agents for more complicated analytic and synthetic tasks. Machines cannot, however, offer the humane solicitude embodied in the ancient nursing watchwords of "tender loving care." They might conceivably free staff members to extend such sought ministrations, although there is as yet no indication that this is in fact what happens under partially automated monitoring.

Sophisticated information processing may exert its most powerful force in the type of complex social epidemiology sketched in Chapters 6 through 8. Researchers are becoming convinced that the major chronic illnesses are subtle and multidetermined. If this is so, our knowledge of causation seems bound to depend on a patient fitting-together of wide ranges of information, from biological indices to facets of social and psychological experience. To tease out configurations from these many bits of knowledge, the researcher needs the means of massing and collating data that constitute the chief virtues of the computer. Physiological monitoring, moreover, may enable investigators to link bodily happenings ever more surely to the multitude of events occurring in the individual's life space. For example, recent evidence from studies of occupational health demonstrates close relations between organic processes and social situations. (Responsible ground personnel at space launchings have been found to exhibit acceleration of pulse rate exceeding that of astronauts themselves.)

The explosion of knowledge represented by automation and information processing is only one striking instance of medicine's ready response to scientific change. It is more than matched by the possibilities inherent in new biological knowledge, fresh understandings of human behavior, and advances in surgical technique. In the main, all of these innovations portend a greatly increased medical capability to affect men's health—and their lives. Man can make and shape himself ever more potently, and in so doing he inevitably confronts a series of grave choices. These choices are not only those of intelligence and rational strategy but also, emphatically, choices of morality and the deepest reaches of human valuing.

Astonishing advances in biology and genetics have brought much more information about the cellular stuff of life. The "coding" of DNA and its progressive untangling means that the door has swung open on our potential ability to influence human characteristics. Whether or not medical science is genuinely in a position to "create" life is a moot point, but there seems to be little doubt that we have started down the road that can lead to profound abilities to alter individual potentialities. These abilities, if consummated, will raise perfectly obvious but presently unanswerable questions: Who is to determine the desired patternings of human characteristics? On what basis of moral value shall such determinations be founded? What modes of social control will be devised to sanction the ultimate in what Erving Goffman called "the tinkering trades"? (Who will guard the tinkerers?)

Similar root queries must be directed to the health professional's use of the emerging possibilities in the behavioral sciences, especially as these intersect with neurophysiology. The drug therapies, for instance, already afford therapists an opportunity to induce substantial behavioral changes. In treatment of the mental illnesses, they have clearly proved enormously beneficial, stabilizing individual personalities and aiding renewed functional effectiveness. Yet chemotherapy is open to abuse at some times and by some criteria of value. Imagine, if one will, a tranquilized Vincent Van Gogh, and try to balance his torment

against his comfort, his furious art against his other human satis-
factions. If experimental work on the electrical stimulation of
areas of the brain comes to fruition, certain behaviors may be
triggered or dampened by electrical impulse. To envision a corti-
cal version of the pacemaker that now stabilizes the heart's con-
tractive ability is perhaps not utterly fantastic. Chemotherapy,
remote stimulation, and so on, are not the bogeymen of perverted
science fiction; they represent devices that may greatly enlarge
man's area of discretion and control, his proficiency in managing
his own and others' behavior. Hence, they promise almost incon-
ceivable advantages in the promotion of health, and at the same
time stir questioning about the health agent's legitimate sphere
of decision. Unless the domain of medicine is to be construed as
limitless, technological and accompanying social change will
surely raise the issue of proper boundaries between those things
that are to be determined by "health" criteria in any narrow
sense and those determined by varieties of other, overlapping
criteria in legal, religious, political, or aesthetic sectors.

For the most part, changes in surgical and allied techniques
for repairing the damage occasioned by the stress of life have
been welcomed by health professionals and laymen: individual
existence can be retrieved, strengthened, lengthened. The virtu-
osity and technical elegance that buttress the effort to preserve
and prolong life do not, however, imply any forthright solutions
to problems of cost, priority, and the minimal dignities of continued tracery of steps in the dance of life. At some juncture, perhaps, even the richest society may be forced to choose among
expenditures: How many aged lives shall be sustained (when all,
perhaps, technically *can* be) in a cost comparison with nurturing
the disadvantaged young?

Already, in the popular press and the councils of Congress,
the United States is being confronted with the decisions implicit
in techniques of organ transplant. Until organs can be successfully fabricated, the supply of healthy organs will presumably
fall far behind the demand. Decay in hearts and kidneys will
occur at a rate outstripping untimely death (in the case of
hearts) or timely donorship (in the case of kidneys) among the
young and vigorous. The resulting moral conundrums scarcely
require comment. In the most vulgar terms: Who is to get whose,
and how are the ranks on waiting lists to be assigned? When is a

young patient conclusively doomed and thus a candidate for heart donorship? In which instances does or does not an aged Nobel laureate outrank a young mechanic on a priority schedule for a new heart or kidney?

Increasingly often, both relatives and more detached observers express concern about the prolongation of life in cases where the patient is more vegetable than animal. General social consensus and medical judgment are agreed that any life is worth saving. The hard questions arise when we specify how long, in what state of "life," and at what economic and human expense. The issue is no longer couched in the traditional terms of arguments about euthanasia because few advocate deliberate induction of death. Rather, debate hinges on how many resources should be devoted to sustaining life in cases when there is no apparent hope that recovery or even minimally competent maintenance is possible. In a sense, of course, withdrawal of massive therapeutic efforts is equivalent to a decision that death is, if not desirable, at least allowable. There is a vast difference between the extraordinary concentration of Soviet medical firepower on a renowned physicist who had been thought fatally injured but was somehow sustained ("the man they would not let die") and the usual treatment of individuals in any society. As medical technique grows ever more proficient, the grounds of choice in such cases will become more stringent. One might well contend that the "natural course" of illness and dying is less and less truly natural and increasingly often a matter of complex decision by healing agents.

If technological-scientific changes are thus shifting the dimensions of judgment in medical research and care, then rapid alterations in social values and strategies are also reshaping the organization of that care. Social values are pressing toward a more equitable distribution of life—and health—chances. This pressure for universal availability of care entails innovation in the methods of delivery and the design of facilities. Facilities are geared to greater openness, easier permeability by various population groups. Intensive efforts are being made to bring delivery closer to the point of most convenience for clients. Moreover, the trend is to experiment with the agents of care, utilizing where feasible health auxiliaries who are themselves members or near members of the client's milieu. The underlying thrust of medical care organization is to embed the helping services more firmly in the community, through literal geographic proximity, through recruitment of health auxiliaries, and above all, through the involvement of wider, representative segments of the population in planning and offering care.

As we noted, particularly in Chapters 3 through 5, health has become part of the domain of public policy as never before. The health future will be marked by the continued definition of health problems as a major national concern and the continued broadening of responsibility for health action. Our contention that the United States may appropriately be termed a "helping society" is clearly borne out by Ward Darley and Anne R. Somers:

> In the Census Bureau categories, health services ranked as the third largest industry in the nation in 1960, exceeded only by agriculture and construction. Its amazing growth between 1950 and 1960 was 54 per cent . . . the rate of increase was twice that for population growth. Projections indicate that either health services or education will be the nation's largest consumer of manpower by 1970.[2]

The sheer bulk of society's energies devoted to health is impressive testimony to our general concern. The concentration on health and education combined also serves to confirm Talcott Parsons' assertion that these are the twin "enabling resources" in an open, competitive society and, further, that a basic decision has been made to enable a far larger proportion of the population than has ever been true in the past.

In an effort to cope with the implications of change, the social organization of health care will be quite drastically realigned. Two primary mechanisms for this realignment are now emerging: planning and community involvement. Although the processes of planning and the processes for widening the base of decision are conceptually distinct, they are closely paired in the health world. Planning is really enforced by the rate and breadth of change. The temporarily expedient or merely reactive approach to health problems is demonstrably inadequate because

[2] W. Darley and A. R. Somers, "Medicine, Money and Manpower— The Challenge to Professional Education. III. Increasing Personnel." *New England Journal of Medicine,* 276 (June 22, 1967), 1414–1423.

today's solutions are quickly made obsolete. Continuous monitoring and projections of future needs and facilities afford the only hope of any community's not being outdistanced (or outflanked) by demands. Drawing a variety of professionals and laymen into the planning process seems inevitable on at least two counts: comprehensive decisions—setting priorities and anticipating patterned needs—require an array of talents and interests, and the carrying out of plans rests not on authoritative directive but on a congeries of choices and interactions among agencies and individuals. Field experience, as well as social psychological experiment, dictates that those who must act in certain ways will do so more effectively and more willingly if they have themselves been parties to the choices that generate action.

Granted that plans are intrinsic to the provision of superior health care and that they must be devised on the basis of multilateral consent, our society is still in a very early stage of social invention, of discovering how these desired strategies are to be accomplished. Indeed, the ferment of ideas in this area of American life is a matter of remarkable excitement and promise. Setting priorities in health planning is an activity that drives us to examine basic values and moral assumptions, paralleling the issues rehearsed earlier in connection with changes in scientific technology. Because not even the richest society can do everything at once, we are faced with hard choices both within health itself and between health needs and various other social needs.

Within health, the competition for resources is pointedly exemplified by George James:

> How easy it is to be dazzled by the saving of a life in a brilliant six-hour surgical operation, and to forget that in Mississippi every day Negro mothers delivering their babies have *six times* the likelihood of dying in the process as the average American white woman.[3]

Perhaps few alternative uses of health money and manpower can be as starkly posed as this. But the *type* of issue persists and has led to ingenious search for some index upon which competing needs might be compared. Marshall W. Raffel sets the problem as follows:

[3] George James, Keynote Address. Third National Conference on Public Health Training (Washington, D.C., August 17, 1967).

Gorham asks one of Government's toughest questions, "How to allocate resources among different competing objectives?" He correctly points out that "tradition and politics, or the categorical imperatives of the moment or age, have governed these allocations."

        *   *   *

The search for some objective measure common to competing social needs is inviting to those seeking a base for resource allocation which can be described as more rational.[4]

Raffel goes on to suggest that one such measure might be "disability days." He proposes that any day on which any individual cannot function effectively in his social role(s) may be construed as a deficit to the society. An index of this sort is obviously subject to hazards of definition, notably in fixing the degree of impairment necessary to qualify a day as one of disability. Raffel notes, however, that priorities might be assigned in accord with the quality or quantity of impairment produced by different health needs and, further, that his concept of disability days might also be applied to alternative education or welfare demands. However reached, choices among priorities lie at the heart of the planning process and hence at the shadowy edge of the health future.

If planning is difficult in itself, mobilizing communities to participate in a comprehensive scheme for health is equally challenging. A rather interesting effort to foster community action was the enterprise of the National Commission on Community Health Services. The commission urged cities of varying sizes throughout the country to undertake "self-studies" in which committees of lay and professional leaders assessed local needs and then composed a plan for meeting them. Moderate success in this process appeared to hinge on the quality of local staff (especially the study staff director's knowledge of community institutions and his ability to communicate persuasively) and the tradition of local problem-solving leadership.[5] Those who try to stimulate

---

[4] Marshall W. Raffel, "Competing Social Needs and the Search for a Common Denominator" (unpublished draft manuscript, January 15, 1968).

[5] A fuller account of these studies is given in Robert N. Wilson, *Community Structure and Health Action* (Washington, D.C.: Public Affairs Press, 1968).

wide population concern about health, a sense of commitment that induces people to act, are still unsure about who to involve, how and when to bring them in, and how to coordinate the welter of existing health agencies. On the topic of community organization, as on so many others, our creativity in social relationships lags far behind our creativity in the physical and natural sciences. Probably the most promising implication for the future lies not in our presently feeble knowledge of how to arrange social patterns to meet health imperatives but in the mood of conscious social experiment that opens the possibility of uncovering such knowledge.

In the last third of the twentieth century, technical medical advances will be joined to a more sophisticated social epidemiology and an experimental health planning in an assault on two major problems. These problems are, first, the alleviation of chronic disease, and second, the vigorous pursuit of positive health through early preventive measures. It seems likely that some concept of efficacy or functional ability in individual performance will be at the core of thought and action in each instance. The fact that chronic illness is and will be very widespread among populations but that mortality is relatively low means that people must be helped to sustain reasonable ways of life despite the fact of persistent handicap. In Albert Camus' phrase, the important thing will be "to live with one's ailments," to maintain a going concern. The emphasis must inevitably come to be placed on capitalizing upon the individual's assets, on encouraging continued function up to the irreducible limit of disability. Living with chronicity, of course, cannot be a matter solely of balancing the individual's strengths and weaknesses in abstraction from the social situations in which he is immersed. Rather, the chronically ill person must be viewed in his repertory of social roles; his configuration of capacities has to be interlocked with the varying demands others will place on him. Thus the alleviation of chronicity depends both on a comprehensive evaluation of the individual's functional capacity *and* on close attention to the social system in its potential for cushioning or exacerbating his flawed abilities.

The quest for health as a state of positive well-being may in the future be translated from a guiding ideal into increasingly tangible preventive strategies. We may move more decisively into a serious attempt to foster competent behavior. One facet of the planning process is surely that of planning for health and against illness. To plan for health means to cultivate in individuals a capacity for satisfying living in the social role networks they inhabit. Here again, the stress will be on competence in such roles as the occupational and familial, rather than solely on maintaining a symptom-free existence "for its own sake." The schools may well become a paramount focus in the fostering of health because they constitute an early stage in the life arc when many disabilities have not yet hardened into persistent handicap. Too, if education for competent living attains the central importance we have assumed, the school will be a vital arena of establishing and grooming effective social role behavior. If change is indeed to be the dominant theme of this society's future, one might guess that good health will be intimately related to the person's capacity for living with change, for maintaining a balanced flexibility in coping with a variety of evolving social expectations.

Bibliography: Selected Introductory Readings

Burling, Temple, Edith M. Lentz, and Robert N. Wilson. *The Give and Take in Hospitals*. New York: Putnam, 1956. One of the first full-scale studies of the human organization of the general hospital. This book examines the various professions and vocations making up a hospital staff, and the relations among the myriad departments involved in patient care. It is an attempt to view the hospital as a unique social system.

Cassel, John, Ralph Patrick, and David Jenkins. "Epidemiological Analysis of the Health Implications of Culture Change: A Conceptual Model," *Annals of the New York Academy of Sciences*, Vol. 84, Art. 17 (December 8, 1960), pp. 938–949. Many of the basic assumptions of modern social epidemiology set forth in brief compass. The article presents a telling argument for the inclusion of social and cultural systems in the quest for the causes of illness, especially in the case of chronic diseases. Specific attention is given to cultural change as it affects whether a man's life course will be one of sickness or health.

Caudill, William. *Effects of Social and Cultural Systems in Reactions to Stress*. Social Science Research Council, Pamphlet No. 14. New York, 1958. An exceptionally lucid discussion of "linked open systems" in the etiology of disease. Caudill demonstrates the utility of a systematic model of cause, drawing on convincing examples of the interpenetration of biological, psychological, and social levels of organization.

Caudill, William. *The Psychiatric Hospital as a Small Society*. The Commonwealth Fund. Cambridge Mass.: Harvard University Press, 1958. A shrewd, stimulating look at a small mental hospital from the inside. The author traces the varied perceptions of patients and staff members, showing how their different attitudes shape the course of therapy. It is a cogent analysis of the effects of formal hospital organization on individual behavior.

Clausen, John A. and Robert Straus, eds. *Medicine and Society. The Annals of the American Academy of Political and Social Science,* Vol. 346 (March 1963). An excellent overview of primary concerns in the field of medical sociology. The authors group their treatments under the general headings of perspectives on medicine and society, the organization of medical resources, education for the health professions, and health and human behavior. Separate articles are especially marked by the incisiveness with which they present research and policy issues.

Dobzhansky, Theodosius. *Mankind Evolving.* New Haven: Yale University Press, 1962. An eminent biologist's summing-up of the biological nature of man. Especially valuable is the interweaving of genetic evidence with aspects of man's psychological and social experience. The author's complex view of the determination of human characteristics—including health —encourages a sophisticated model of cause.

Freeman, Howard E., Sol Levine, and Leo G. Reeder. *Handbook of Medical Sociology.* Englewood Cliffs, N.J.: Prentice-Hall, 1963. A comprehensive survey of the state of the art of medical sociology. The separate topical chapters are, in general, reliable and incisive. Especially notable is the range of references and the thorough bibliography of the field prepared by Ozzie G. Simmons.

Galdston, Iago. *The Meaning of Social Medicine.* The Commonwealth Fund. Cambridge, Mass.: Harvard University Press, 1954. A provocative, challenging statement that supports a preventive and life-enhancing approach to health care, as contrasted to the traditional focus on specific cures. Dr. Galdston argues that we have exchanged high mortality for high morbidity, saving people from death, yet not making them well. The argument contains significant implications for medical education.

Goffman, Erving. *Asylums.* Garden City, N.Y.: Doubleday, 1961. An absorbing account of mental hospitalization, featuring, at close observation, an analysis of the patient's career. The author traces the process by which a large mental hospital, as exemplar of a "total institution," shapes patient behavior and personality expression. The institution, rather than the predisposing illness, is seen as the chief determinant of patient adaptation.

Halliday, James L. *Psychosocial Medicine*. New York: Norton, 1948. A stimulating, audacious application of the concepts of psychosomatic medicine to population groups. The author asserts that modern medicine must become increasingly concerned with the psychological environment as a cause of ill health. He further contends that contemporary society is "sick," and that this sickness is reflected in the rising incidence of psychosomatic and psychiatric diseases.

Health Is a Community Affair. Report of the National Commission on Community Health Services. Cambridge, Mass.: Harvard University Press, 1967. A volume devoted to the planning of health care in American communities. The report makes recommendations for action in a number of personal and environmental health problems. Emphasis is placed on local planning, with the involvement of a broad base of concerned citizens.

Hollingshead, August B., and Frederick C. Redlich. *Social Class and Mental Illness*. New York: Wiley, 1958. A documentation of the mental health disadvantages of the economically impoverished. A landmark of social psychiatric research, this study shows that not only do those lowest in the community's social scale have heightened rates of some of the most disabling psychoses, but they also receive less favored modes of treatment and have longer hospital stays than do people of higher social status.

Jahoda, Marie. *Current Criteria of Positive Mental Health*. New York: Basic Books, 1958. A superior synthesis of the leading ideas about psychological health. Dr. Jahoda construes health as more than the absence of disabling symptoms; she sees it as a positive state of maturity and wholeness of personality. This fine contribution to a concept of healthful living has important implications for preventive medicine.

Johnson, Albert L., C. David Jenkins, Ralph Patrick, and Travis J. Northcutt, Jr. *Epidemiology of Polio Vaccine Acceptance*. Florida State Board of Health. Monograph Number 3, 1962. A brilliant investigation of the factors influencing peoples' responses to a health program. The authors, in two extensive field surveys, uncover the characteristics of takers and non-takers of free polio vaccine. This monograph not only identifies social class and ethnic differences in the respondents, but also suggests techniques for increasing the response of hard-to-reach groups.

Leighton, Alexander H. *My Name Is Legion*. New York: Basic Books, 1959. One of the most ambitious and intelligent attempts to develop a framework for the social etiology of psychological disorder. This and succeeding volumes of the Stirling County Study seek to link the dynamics of individual illness to the community matrix of life experience. The study is especially original in its articulation of community organization and levels of psychiatric symptoms in the population.

Leighton, Alexander H., John A. Clausen, and Robert N. Wilson, eds. *Explorations in Social Psychiatry*. New York: Basic Books, 1957. A multi-discipline approach to the social origins and consequences of psychological disorder. The several authors move from a consideration of familial experience in the genesis of individual illness to the broad implications for the community of the prevalence of mental illness. The editors identify major theoretical issues in social psychiatry and relate these to the varied particular contributions.

Lerner, Monroe, and Odin W. Anderson. *Health Progress in the United States, 1900–1960*. Chicago: The University of Chicago Press, 1963. A significant assessment of the state of health of the American population. By summarizing rates of illness in different sectors of society, the authors offer a basis for causal hypotheses. Major interest inheres in the description of changing patterns of illness in the United States during the twentieth century.

Marti-Ibanez, Felix, ed. *Sigerist on the History of Medicine*. New York: M.D. Publications, 1960. Roemer, Milton I., ed. *Sigerist on the Sociology of Medicine*. New York: M.D. Publications, Inc., 1960. Two collections of papers by the late Henry E. Sigerist that are a mine of historical information, sociological insight, and, above all, humanistic delight. Treating medicine as a human enterprise grounded in particular personalities and social settings, Sigerist roams widely and perceptively through the story of man's encounters with illness and his strivings for health.

Merton, Robert K., George G. Reader and Patricia L. Kendall, eds. The Commonwealth Fund. *The Student-Physician: Introductory Studies in the Sociology of Medical Education.* Cambridge, Mass.: Harvard University Press, 1957. A report on a series of investigations into the process of becoming a physician. The authors look closely at three leading medical schools, asking how students choose a medical career, how they learn to enact professional roles, and how they accumulate attitudes and values as well as technical medical knowledge. The volume includes a superb historical and theoretical essay by Robert K. Merton.

Parsons, Talcott. *The Social System.* New York: Free Press, 1951, pp. 428–73. A classic analysis of American medical practice as a social system and as part of the larger context of United States society. Especially notable for its standard, ideal-typical formulation of the social roles of patient and physician, its description of the sick role has been very influential in research on patient behavior.

Paul, Benjamin D., ed. *Health, Culture, and Community.* New York: Russell Sage Foundation, 1955. The pioneering effort to assess problems of introducing health programs into diverse cultural settings. This volume is marked by the editor's sophisticated application of social scientific analysis to public health practice. Presentation of specific case materials lends immediacy to the theoretical principles.

Saunders, Lyle. *Cultural Difference and Medical Care.* New York: Russell Sage Foundation, 1954. A thoughtful examination of the problems entailed in the practice of modern medicine among Spanish-speaking people in the southwestern United States. Using cogent field observations, Saunders analyzes Latin culture and Anglo health professionals to find the elements that make communication—and treatment—difficult.

Simmons, Leo W., and Harold G. Wolff. *Social Science in Medicine*. New York: Russell Sage Foundation, 1954. One of the earliest attempts to lay down a conceptual underpinning for the social scientist's approach to medical problems. The authors are persuasive in their analysis of the links among sociocultural systems, the concept of stress, and the etiology of disease.

Skipper, James K., and Robert C. Leonard, eds. *Social Interaction and Patient Care*. Philadelphia: Lippincott, 1965. The work of many hands, a volume centering on processes of communication in health care. The social psychology of care-giving is viewed in terms of interaction between helper and helped. It is remarkable for the many demonstrations of the proposition that human factors in treatment may be as important as strictly medical or surgical intervention.

Index

A Note on the Type

The text of this book was set in Caledonia, a Linotype face designed by W. A. Dwiggins. It belongs to the family of printing types called "modern face" by printers—a term used to mark the change in style of type letters that occurred about 1800. Caledonia borders on the general design of Scotch Modern, but is more freely drawn than that letter.